Internet Guide
to Herbal Remedies

THE HAWORTH INFORMATION PRESS®
Haworth Internet Medical Guides
M. Sandra Wood, MLS
Editor

The Guide to Complementary and Alternative Medicine on the Internet by Lillian R. Brazin

Internet Guide to Travel Health by Elizabeth Connor

Internet Guide to Food Safety and Security by Elizabeth Connor

Internet Guide to Cosmetic Surgery for Women by M. Sandra Wood

Internet Guide to Anti-Aging and Longevity by Elizabeth Connor

Internet Guide to Herbal Remedies by David J. Owen

Internet Guide to Medical Diets and Nutrition by Lillian R. Brazin

Internet Guide to Cosmetic Surgery for Men by M. Sandra Wood

Internet Resources on Obesity by Lillian R. Brazin

Internet Guide
to Herbal Remedies

David J. Owen, MA, PhD

The Haworth Information Press®
An Imprint of The Haworth Press
New York • London • Oxford

For more information on this book or to order, visit
http://www.haworthpress.com/store/product.asp?sku=5855

or call 1-800-HAWORTH (800-429-6784) in the United States and Canada
or (607) 722-5857 outside the United States and Canada

or contact orders@HaworthPress.com

Published by

The Haworth Information Press®, an imprint of The Haworth Press, Inc., 10 Alice Street, Binghamton, NY 13904-1580.

PUBLISHER'S NOTE
The development, preparation, and publication of this work has been undertaken with great care. However, the Publisher, employees, editors, and agents of The Haworth Press are not responsible for any errors contained herein or for consequences that may ensue from use of materials or information contained in this work. The Haworth Press is committed to the dissemination of ideas and information according to the highest standards of intellectual freedom and the free exchange of ideas. Statements made and opinions expressed in this publication do not necessarily reflect the views of the Publisher, Directors, management, or staff of The Haworth Press, Inc., or an endorsement by them.

Due to the ever-changing nature of the Internet, Web site names and addresses, though verified to the best of the publisher's ability, should not be accepted as accurate without independent verification.

Cover design by Kerry E. Mack.

Library of Congress Cataloging-in-Publication Data

Owen, David J.
    Internet guide to herbal remedies / David J. Owen.
        p. cm.
    Includes bibliographical references and index.
    ISBN-13: 978-0-7890-2230-1 (case-13 : alk. paper)
    ISBN-13: 978-0-7890-2231-8 (soft-13 : alk. paper)
    ISBN-10: 0-7890-2230-3 (case-10 : alk. paper)
    ISBN-10: 0-7890-2231-1 (soft-10 : alk. paper)
    1. Herbs—Therapeutic use—Computer network resources—Directories. 2. Web sites—Directories. I. Title.

    RM666.H33O976 2006
    025.06'615321—dc22

                                                                2006015772

To the memory of my mother and to the memory
of my mentor, Miss Margaret "Maggie" Collins

NOTES FOR PROFESSIONAL LIBRARIANS AND LIBRARY USERS

This is an original book title published by The Haworth Information Press®, an imprint of The Haworth Press, Inc. Unless otherwise noted in specific chapters with attribution, materials in this book have not been previously published elsewhere in any format or language.

CONSERVATION AND PRESERVATION NOTES

All books published by The Haworth Press, Inc., and its imprints are printed on certified pH neutral, acid-free book grade paper. This paper meets the minimum requirements of American National Standard for Information Sciences-Permanence of Paper for Printed Material, ANSI Z39.48-1984.

DIGITAL OBJECT IDENTIFIER (DOI) LINKING

The Haworth Press is participating in reference linking for elements of our original books. (For more information on reference linking initiatives, please consult the CrossRef Web site at www.crossref.org.) When citing an element of this book such as a chapter, include the element's Digital Object Identifier (DOI) as the last item of the reference. A Digital Object Identifier is a persistent, authoritative, and unique identifier that a publisher assigns to each element of a book. Because of its persistence, DOIs will enable The Haworth Press and other publishers to link to the element referenced, and the link will not break over time. This will be a great resource in scholarly research.

CONTENTS

ABOUT THE AUTHOR

David J. Owen, MA, PhD, is Education Coordinator for the Basic Sciences in the Library and Center for Knowledge Management at the University of California, San Francisco. He also holds an appointment as Assistant Clinical Professor in the UCSF School of Pharmacy. Dr. Owen previously worked as an information specialist in the biotechnology field and is the author of *The Herbal Internet Companion: Herbs and Herbal Medicine Online* (Haworth).

Acknowledgments

This book would have taken longer to complete without an award from the University-wide Research Grants for Librarians program provided by the Librarians Association of the University of California (LAUC). This grant allowed me to spend some time away from the library during 2004-2005 to concentrate on the actual writing.

I wish to acknowledge the following people who, in many different ways, provided support and encouragement during the writing of this book: Mr. Stephen Rosenberg, Ben, Andy, Keith, David, and Warren; my friend and colleague Min-Lin Fang; my dad and my sister Christine. Thanks also to M. Sandra Wood and the staff at The Haworth Press.

Internet Guide to Herbal Remedies
© 2006 by The Haworth Press, Inc. All rights reserved.
doi:10.1300/5855_a

Introduction

The next best thing to knowing something is knowing where to find it.

Samuel Johnson

This book is aimed at the consumer who wishes to go online and find reliable information on herbs and herbal remedies. Though information about herbs is widely available on the Internet, its quality is very uneven and, in my opinion, much of it is of little value to the average user. Many health-related Web sites do provide accurate and up-to-date news, facts, and advice about herbs, but many others do not. Instead, they may provide information that is not only misleading, but possibly harmful. Literally thousands of Web sites are dedicated to nearly every conceivable health subject. How do you find the good stuff? Which Web sites can you trust? How do you know when information is misleading or when a Web site is just a thinly veiled advertisement for someone selling a product? If you are new to using the Internet to find health information, or are an experienced surfer wishing to find herbal information you can trust, this book can help you.

My first encounter with medicinal herbs occurred in England during my student days in the 1970s, when the "back to nature" movement rekindled public interest in so-called "alternative" medical remedies. Out of curiosity, and in a search for something to treat insomnia, I picked up a copy of Maud Grieve's 1931 *A Modern Herbal*[1] in a secondhand book store.* Among the many delights and revelations in this book was a

---

*Mrs. Grieve's *Modern Herbal* was published in 1931 and at the time was considered "modern" because it was the first new herbal for over 100 years. Though still widely used by herbalists, it's rather dated now and is mainly of historical interest.

chapter on the benefits of valerian tea as a way to get a good night's sleep. At that time you couldn't buy herbal preparations at your local pharmacy, so off I trotted to an old dusty herbal shop buried away in a London suburb, where both the shop and its owner seemed to have stepped straight out of a Charles Dickens novel. Valerian proved to be an effective remedy for getting to sleep at night and many years later I still occasionally use it, along with cups of mint tea to perk up during the day and chamomile for relaxation after a hard day's work.

Much has changed in the herbal world since the 1970s. On my last visit to England I found a whole section of shelves in my parents' local supermarket devoted entirely to herbal teas. In addition to the usual favorites such as mint and chamomile, I discovered teas containing licorice, raspberry, new ones such as chi (pronounced like "pie") and some I'd never heard of, such as "red tea" or rooibos (pronounced ROY-boss), a tea with high levels of antioxidants. In the town's main pharmacy, next to shelves filled with the standard drugs such as aspirin, cough medicines, and antibiotic cream, I discovered a wide range of herbal products that wouldn't have been there a decade ago: St. John's wort for depression, echinacea for insomnia, and tea tree antiseptic oil for fungal infections.

Herbs are currently enjoying an unprecedented popularity: see Table I.1 for a list of the most popular ones used in the United States. Although herbal remedies have been prescribed by physicians in several European countries for many years, the rapid rise of interest in so-called "alternative therapies" by the American public has taken many health professionals in the United States completely by surprise. It was only in the 1990s that they really became aware of just how many of their patients actually use them. Until recently, there was a limited number of professional handbooks and consumer guides: even physicians had a hard job finding information. Fortunately, mainstream medicine is becoming more open-minded about herbs, acupuncture, and other unconventional therapies, so many health care providers are now much better informed than they used to be. Furthermore, many more scientific studies are now being carried out on popular herbs such as echinacea and St. John's wort, and federal agencies such as the National Center for Complementary and Alternative Medicine (NCCAM) have been set up to make information more readily available to the public.

TABLE I.1. Most Popular Herbs Sold in the United States.

Common Name	Scientific Name	Used For
Ginkgo	*Ginkgo biloba*	Dementia
St. John's wort	*Hypericum perforatum*	Depression
Ginseng	*Panax ginseng*	Fatigue and weakness
Garlic	*Allium sativum*	High cholesterol
Echinacea	*Echinacea pupurea*	Colds
Saw palmetto	*Serenoa repens*	Prostate conditions
Kava kava	*Piper methysticum*	Anxiety
Valerian	*Valeriana officinalis*	Insomnia
Evening primrose	*Oenothera macrocarpa*	Inflammation
Goldenseal	*Hydrastis canadensis*	Colds
Milk thistle	*Silybum marianum*	Liver disorders
Bilbery	*Vaccinium myrtillus*	Eye disorders
Black cohosh	*Cimicifuga racemosa*	Menopause, premenstrual syndrome
Cranberry	*Vaccinium macrocarpon*	Urinary tract infections

It seems somewhat ironic that the resurgence of public interest in medical practices once widely regarded as relics of more ignorant times should have occurred at a time when computers and the Internet are revolutionizing the way we access and use information. An increasing number of people are now seeking health information online. Information that used to be only available in research journals or in the collection of a local medical library is now being published on Web sites that can be accessed by anyone with a home computer and an Internet Service Provider (ISP). However, many health professionals and organizations are justifiably concerned about consumers using the Internet to find health information because of the extreme variability in its quality. Casually surfing the Web for herbal information is not recommended, since you'll have to navigate a tangled maze of unsubstantiated claims, anecdotal information, and a good deal of mumbo jumbo, a large percentage of it written by nonprofessionals or herbal product manufacturers. Some of this information is often more confusing than helpful, with seemingly contradictory conclusions on whether a particular herb is really effective.

This book is intended to guide you to the best online resources for herbal information. Though the main focus is on Web sites, it describes search tools, newsgroups, LISTSERVs, chat rooms, and databases that will be of help to anyone seeking up-to-date information. This book not only tells you where to find the good stuff, but also includes tips to make you a better "surfer." Although its focus is on Web sites where you can go to find advice on the safety, use, and effectiveness of herbal remedies, I have also included chapters on issues that I think are of importance to anyone who wishes to have a better understanding of herbal medicine in the United States. Issues include current laws and regulations governing herbal use and the twin problems of fraud and quackery. There's also a little basic botany included, since you'll find it helpful to know something about how herbs are named and which parts of the plant are used. Since alternative therapies are increasingly being used by vets and pet owners, I've not ignored Fluffy the cat and Spot the dog, and have included Web sites for pet owners.

My choice of Web sites may seem biased toward those affiliated with government agencies or university medical centers. This is simply because government or university-run Web sites are among the best sources for scientifically sound health and medical information. Private practitioners or not-for-profit organizations may have marketing, social, or political agendas that can influence the type of information they provide. Furthermore, and perhaps more important, we often know very little about the safety and effectiveness of many herbal remedies currently on the market. Many unscrupulous individuals are exploiting this ignorance to promote unproven and sometimes dangerous remedies to an unsuspecting public. So I believe it is best to err on the side of caution. Similarly, several well-known herbal Web sites set up by individuals or organizations have been excluded, for though they may be an excellent source of information for the experienced and knowledgeable user, they are not really suitable for the average consumer wishing to find out if he or she should use echinacea to fight a cold (refer to my other book if you wish to consult a more comprehensive review of herbal Web sites: *The Herbal Internet Companion: Herbs and Herbal Medicine Online*[2]). This is not necessarily a reflection of the quality of the information or the people or organizations providing it.

Good, reliable information is out there on the Internet if you know where to find it. It's a wonderful resource if you keep your wits about you. Always remember, however, that any information you find should be discussed with your doctor or other health care provider.

NOTES

1. Grieve, M. *A Modern Herbal; the Medicinal, Culinary, Cosmetic and Economic Properties, Cultivation and Folk-Lore of Herbs, Grasses, Fungi, Shrubs & Trees with All Their Modern Scientific Uses.* New York: Dover Publications; 1971.
2. Owen, D. *The Herbal Internet Companian: Herbs and Herbal Medicine Online.* Binghamton, NY: The Haworth Press; 2002.

Chapter 1

Navigating the World Wide Web

When I took office, only high energy physicists had ever heard of
what is called the World Wide Web . . . now even my cat has its
own page.

Bill Clinton

This chapter will go over some of the things you need to know about
the Internet and the World Wide Web, so you can get the most out of going online. Keep in mind that the Web is only part of the Internet,
though it's the most useful part for finding herbal information. We'll
cover chat rooms, electronic discussion groups, and newsgroups in a
later chapter.

One of the most frustrating things about the Web is that it has become so BIG! There is so much there, both good and bad, and finding
reliable information can be a challenge. It's often difficult for people to
grasp just how big it really is, and in fact no one is really quite sure. Recently, Yahoo! claimed that its search engine indexes over 19 billion
documents.[1] If that figure doesn't mean much to you, don't worry, because however big it really is, it's *enormous,* and it means that trying to
find good information can be like looking for that needle in a haystack.

UNDERSTANDING WEB ADDRESSES

The World Wide Web (www), or simply the Web, is a huge worldwide network of computers that exchange information, such as text,

Internet Guide to Herbal Remedies
© 2006 by The Haworth Press, Inc. All rights reserved.
doi:10.1300/5855_02

pictures, and sound. These computers talk to one other using the Internet. If you looked at a map of the Internet it would look like a huge tangled spider's web, which is where the name for the World Wide Web comes from. It's important to know that each page on the Web has a location, and its location is indicated by a Web address. The address tells the computer exactly where this page can be found, just as your home address tells someone where you can be found. This Web address is called the uniform resource locator (URL).

Each Web-accessible document has a unique URL that can be used to pull it up on your Web browser. You may see the address of the document you're currently viewing in the Address box in the Internet Explorer Address bar. When you move the mouse pointer over links on a page, you'll see the address of the linked documents appear at the bottom of the browser window.

A Web site has one or more related Web pages, depending on how it's designed. These pages are linked together through a system of hyperlinks. A hyperlink is a link from a document that, when clicked, opens another page or file. You can tell when something is a hyperlink to another page: when you move your cursor over a text link or over a graphic link, it will change from an arrow to a hand. Each Web site has a homepage, which can be thought of as the starting point of the site. Homepages are like the table of contents in a book or magazine, usually providing an overview of what you'll find at the site.

You'll find it useful to know a little bit about how a URL acts as an Internet address. Let's take a look at the URL for a handout on St. John's wort, stored on a computer at the Food and Drug Administration (FDA): <http://www.fda.gov/health/stjohnswort.html>.

- The first part of the URL, before the colon (:), identifies the type of document we are dealing with. hypertext transfer protocol (http) is simply a protocol (set of rules) used to retrieve a resource from the Internet. It tells us this is indeed a Web page that will be sent in the format all Web browsers can read. For Web addresses, a second protocol is sometimes widely used: most Web pages are sent across the network "unencrypted." That is, if someone were snooping on you, they could see exactly what you were looking at, or see all the information you might be entering into an online order form. URLs that begin with https, however, are transmitted "encrypted," meaning that someone looking at an http file as it is transferred over the network would see nothing but gibberish. This is obviously a good thing for sensitive information such as user names and passwords, credit card information, and so on.

- The "www.fda.gov" part is the name of the computer where the document is stored. You'll often see www in addresses though this is not really necessary. Obviously, "fda" stands for the Food and Drug Administration. A URL usually uses forward slashes (/) and dots to separate its parts. The ".gov" part is called the "top-level domain" name signifying that it's a U.S. federal government computer. Other options are .com or .net for general commercial Web servers, .edu for servers at higher educational institutions, and .org for nonprofit organizations. Note that Web servers located in other countries end in a two-letter code to identify that country: .uk for the United Kingdom, .fr for France, .de for Germany, .jp for Japan, and so on.
- The "/" tells us we're looking in a directory called "health." The "stjohnswort.html" refers to the specific page, though sometimes the ".html" part is often hidden from you. (Those pesky "Web masters," the people who are in charge of the Web site, are always moving pages around, so if a document has moved places on a Web site you can usually go to the homepage to track it down.) In this case, you could go up through the directory to the homepage at <www.fda.gov>.

You don't need to remember much of the previous discussion to function in today's information society. Just try to remember that a URL is a World Wide Web address and that most Web addresses begin with "http."

BROWSERS

A Web browser, or simply browser, is software that locates and displays Web pages. For example, Microsoft's Internet Explorer (IE) is one of the most commonly used browsers, while Netscape Navigator, Foxfire, and Apple's Safari are used to a lesser extent. Internet Explorer comes preloaded on all computers using Microsoft Windows. You can download browser software for free from each company's Web site (see URLs at the end of this chapter). Note that there are slight differences between the Windows and Macintosh versions.

WEB SURFING WITH "BOOKMARKS" OR "FAVORITES"

One of the best ways to move around the Web is to let your browser remember the address so it's easy to visit it again later. With Internet Explorer you save URLs as "Favorites." When you are on a Web site, select the Favorites menu and click "Add to Favorites." A box will pop up, asking you to name the site. Click OK to add the site to your Favorites. To return to the site later, select the Favorites menu and click on the name of the site in the list. Netscape Navigator calls them "Bookmarks." While you are on the site, select Bookmarks. Next to the Location box, click Add Bookmark. If you would like to edit or rename your bookmarks, choose Edit Bookmarks from the same location.

HOW TO NAVIGATE A WEB SITE

You don't need to be a computer whiz kid in order to move easily around a Web site but knowing a few important things will make it easier for you to find any information that may be buried in the site's pages. The first thing you need to know is that the Back button on your browser is the way to go back a page, and the Forward button is the way to move forward a page. Moving forward and backward is based strictly on pages you've already visited during your current online session. These two buttons are most useful for moving back and forth among two or three pages you're looking at at a given moment. (Exhibit 1.1 shows the most useful Internet Explorer features for moving between Web sites.) Using hyperlinks to move around the Web is like flipping through the pages of a book, moving to an entirely different part of the book, or opening another book altogether. Sometimes it's not obvious which parts of a Web page are hyperlinks. They may be blue underlined words, but they can also be an image on a page. The best way to tell if something on a Web page is a hyperlink is to slide your cursor

EXHIBIT 1.1.
Using Your Browser to Move Around the Web

Back and Forward

| ⇐ Back ▾ ⇒ ▾ | As you move between different Web pages your browser keeps track of where you've been. The toolbar buttons allow you to move backward and forward between pages. |

Stop

Clicking on this allows you to stop the loading of pages or documents. You may want to do this if it is taking too long, or if there is no response from the Web page.

Home

This takes you back to your home page. You can specify which home page to use by going to Internet Options.

Favorites

| ✷ Favorites | This is where you create a list of your favorite sites so you can easily go back to them without having to enter the URL again. |

History

| ✷ History | This provides a history of sites you've visited. |

over it. If it changes from an arrow to a little hand, then you know that it's a hyperlink. If you click when the cursor is a hand, then you'll follow the hyperlink and a new page will appear in your browser.

Most Web sites try to make it easy for you to move from page to page on their site. The homepage usually has a navigation bar prominently displayed to help you find the most important pages, and is usually on the left-hand side or top area of the page. Once you spot a site's main navigation bar, you should be able to go almost anywhere on the site just by clicking on various links. This is a great way to get a quick overview of what a site has to offer and it's also a good way to go straight to your favorite parts of the site on return visits. Look also for a Site Map: this is a map of a Web site's content that allows you to navigate through the site to find the information you're looking for.

If the site has one, read the FAQs (Frequently Asked Questions) first. This document often provides answers to questions commonly asked about the Web site. If all else fails use the site's search engine, essentially a searchable index of the site's pages. Search engines are increasingly being added to individual Web sites to allow users to search the contents of a site.

AVOIDING EYESTRAIN

If you're viewing a Web page and the letters are too small to read, most Web browsers have easy ways to let you enlarge the size of the letters, or fonts. If you are using recent versions of Internet Explorer, you can use the "View" menu and "Text Size" to adjust the font size.

WEB SITES FOR BROWSER DOWNLOADS

The following URLs are sites that allow you to download Internet Explorer, Netscape Navigator, Foxfire, or Safari, with links to tutorials on getting the most out of each browser.

Microsoft (Download Explorer)
<http://www.microsoft.com/>

This Web site is the download page for Internet Explorer.

Netscape (Download Communicator)
<http://channels.netscape.com/ns/browsers/default.jsp>

This Web site is the download page for Netscape Communicator.

Firefox
<http://www.mozilla.org/products/firefox/>

This Web site is the download page for Firefox.

Safari
<http://www.apple.com/safari>

Safari is a Web browser created by Apple Computer made specifically for Apple computers running OS X.

How To Get the Most Out of Internet Explorer
<http://www.microsoft.com/windows/ie/using/howto/ default.mspx>

This site has articles on how to get the most out of using Internet Explorer. Learn the basics for finding Web pages, using Favorites, and more about security and privacy settings.

NOTE

1. Markoff J. Google and Yahoo Bicker Over the Size of Their Turf. *The International Herald Tribune.* August 16, 2005: 13.

Chapter 2

Online Conversations

"If I have a Web log, is it something my doctor should remove?"

One of the great attractions of the Internet is that you can use it to communicate with people around the world and exchange information. Virtual communities and social networks are being created in cyberspace, through mailing lists, newsgroups, electronic discussion forums, Web-based discussion forums, and live chat rooms. The Internet has opened a new social space for communication. An increasing number of health care consumers are now using the Internet for health-related research using newsgroups and chat rooms. These are obviously more casual forms of information gathering than using the Web, so you need to be particularly careful about using any information that someone passes on to you. If you do find something that interests you, see what some of the more reliable Web sites have to say on the topic. If you join health-related discussion lists, usenet groups, or chat rooms, try to find those monitored by a health care practitioner: this will offer protection against the possible sharing of wrong or irrelevant information.

ELECTRONIC DISCUSSION GROUPS

The two oldest forms of online discussion groups are electronic mailing lists and newsgroups. An electronic mailing list, sometimes called a LISTSERV, is a subject-oriented online discussion group that uses e-mail as its primary means of communication. Messages posted

Internet Guide to Herbal Remedies
© 2006 by The Haworth Press, Inc. All rights reserved.
doi:10.1300/5855_03

to a LISTSERV are automatically sent to everyone who has subscribed. Subscribers can actively take part in ongoing discussions, known as "threads," asking questions, answering others' questions, or simply observing—a practice known as "lurking." Once you subscribe, new messages in the form of e-mail are automatically delivered to your electronic mailbox. You can simply read the contents of the messages, you can merely "lurk" in the background and not contribute to the mailing list, or you can ask a question, give your opinion, and participate in an ongoing discussion. Mailing lists can involve just a few people or tens of thousands. Thousands of mailing lists exist covering almost any conceivable health topic.

Usenet newsgroups, sometimes referred to as online forums, are open discussion groups on a wide range of topics where people can contribute to a discussion by leaving a message of interest. LISTSERVs and usenet newsgroups are similar in many respects, but LISTSERVs rely on e-mail as a way to distribute information, whereas usenet functions more like a giant collection of electronic bulletin boards. Newsgroups exist on thousands of topics and are very useful for bringing people together with similar interests. A "newsreader" is software that you need in order to read comments posted in newsgroups. This software is now automatically incorporated into Internet browsers, so usually this is the only program you need to participate in an online discussion. Newsgroups can either be "moderated" (where a message can only be posted with approval) or "open" (where a message can be posted without anyone's approval). The best source on the Web for access to usenet is Google Groups, which allows you to read, search, participate in, and subscribe to discussion forums.

CHAT ROOMS AND INSTANT MESSAGING

A chat room is exactly what it sounds like—a place on the Internet where people with similar interests can chat and socialize. Messages typed in by one user appear instantly to everybody who is in that chat room. Some chat rooms are "moderated," which means not all messages are broadcast because they might be off topic, use bad language, or repeat undesirable messages or ones with obscene language. The majority of chat rooms, however, remain "open," messages are posted automatically with no human intervention. People can often enter a chat room without any verification of who they are. Please remember that anything you type in a chat room can be seen by everyone who is using that chat room, so be careful what you type. Do not give out personal information such as your last name, home address, or telephone number.

You probably already use e-mail, so I'm not going to cover it here. Instant messaging (IM) is a sort of cross between e-mail and a telephone call. It's a fast, convenient, and simple way to communicate with one or more people online in real time. With IMs, you can create a contact list (or "buddy list") and send and receive messages to any or all of them, as long as they are also online. You can customize your buddy lists and share files, photographs, videos, sounds, and Internet links. Unlike e-mail, where there is a time lag, with instant messaging you can have a conversation without any delays.

WEB LOGS

More and more people are now keeping Web logs. A Web log, or "blog" for short, is a diary-style Web site in which the author (a "blogger") posts commentaries and links to other Web pages he or she finds interesting. Web logs are usually created by one person, so they're often very personal. Entries are usually brief and it might be updated every few hours or merely every few days. The universe of Web logs is usually called the "blogosphere." A number of blog-hosting Web sites and services, plus software packages allow people to create their own Web log. Because of the very informal nature of Web logs I don't think you should use them for gathering information on herbal medicines. Some of the ones I've checked either don't have any herbal information you won't find on the reputable Web sites or have been primarily set up to help sell a product. If you want to see what blogs look like go to the Yahoo! Directory and select Health and Medicine.

NETIQUETTE

Effective communication on the Internet is governed by what is known as "netiquette" (Internet etiquette) which refers to rules of behavior governing the use of Internet services, including e-mail, chat, and communicating via discussion groups. Usually when we talk face-to-face with someone, body language, including facial expressions, helps us communicate some things better than words. Subtle messages often pass between us without us being aware of them. On the Internet, body language is missing, so one very useful netiquette tool is the use of emoticons ("smileys") to help express emotion or intent in Internet communication. Emoticons can be used in e-mail, instant messages, and chat messages, and are rather cartoonish in appearance. However, they help get a feeling across when words might be misunderstood. Standard emoticons include:

Expression of humor   ☺
Frown, or expression of sadness   ☹
Wink, or expression of sarcasm   ;-)

WEB SITES FOR CHATTING ONLINE

Yahoo! Directory/Weblogs
<http://dir.yahoo.com/Computers_and_Internet/Internet/World_ Wide_Web/Weblogs/>

Yahoo! Groups
<http://groups.yahoo.com/>

The Health and Wellness section lists over 5,000 newsgroups for Alternative Medicine. Check out the Herbal Medicine section but be careful about using some of the information and advice you may find. Remember that many of these groups are used by herbal product manufacturers to promote their wares.

Yahoo! Chat
\<http://chat.yahoo.com/\>

Fee-based chat rooms.

MSN Chat
\<http://chat.msn.com/\>

Requires a subscription.

MSN Hotmail
\<http://www.msn.com/\>

One of many free e-mail systems on the Internet.

Yahoo! Mail
\<http://mail.yahoo.com/\>

One of many free e-mail systems on the Internet.

Google Groups
\<http://groups.google.com/\>

Google Groups contains the world's most comprehensive archive of usenet postings, dating back to 1981. Click on Groups Help to learn all about using newsgroups.

CataList: the Catalog of LISTSERV® lists
\<http://www.lsoft.com/lists/listref.html\>

A searchable index of public online discussion lists.

Netiquette Home Page
\<http://www.albion.com/netiquette/\>

The core rules of netiquette excerpted from the book *Netiquette* by Virginia Shea.

Yahoo! Directory/Health and Medicine Weblogs
<http://dir.yahoo.com/Computers_and_Internet/Internet/World_Wide_Web/Weblogs/>

Click on Health and Medicine to see a list of available blogs. Check out the Health Facts and Fears blog from the American Council on Science and Health.

REFERENCE

Shea, Virginia. *Netiquette.* San Francisco: Albion Books; 1994.

Chapter 3

Herbal Information on the Internet

Getting information off the Internet is like taking a drink from a fire hydrant.

Mitchell Kapor

THE GOOD, THE BAD, AND THE SALES PITCH

First, the good news: the quality of herbal information available online has improved considerably over the past few years and there are now many Web sites which provide good, reliable information on how to use herbal remedies. Now the bad news: you're unlikely to find any of the best Web sites by simply typing search terms into an Internet search engine such as Google. Using an Internet search engine you'll pull up thousands of Web sites, providing information of extremely variable quality, and if you look very closely at these sites you'll notice that most of them are sponsored by herbal product manufacturers trying to convince you to buy their products—for which they often make extravagant and sometimes false claims! (Nowadays I only use a search engine when I want to find a Web site that I already know exists.)

It's technically very easy and cheap to set up a Web site and this can be done by practically anyone with a computer, inexpensive software, and access to the Internet. Unlike the information you'll find in medical journals, however, there is little regulation or standardization of Web-based information and its quality is often determined solely by the organizations and individuals who publish it. This is of particular concern

Internet Guide to Herbal Remedies
© 2006 by The Haworth Press, Inc. All rights reserved.
doi:10.1300/5855_04

EXHIBIT 3.1.
How to Recognize a Reliable Web Site

Source	Is the site provided by a well-known and respected source?
Content	Where does the information come from? Does it provide evidence to support its claims? Personal testimonials are not evidence.
Disclosure	What is the mission or scope of the site?
Links	Are there links to other high-quality sites?
Design	Is it easy to find the information?
Interactivity	Is their a way for you to contact the author or Web site administrator?
Referral	Does the site encourage you to discuss information with your physician or other health care provider?
Date	When was the information last updated?

because misinformation or the incorrect use of medical information can be harmful. As the American public's interest in herbs grows, so does the number of Web sites containing a large amount of dubious claims and misinformation.

So, how do you go about sorting the good stuff from the bad? Though the chief aim of this book is to direct you to those Web sites that I consider to be some of the best ones around, you'll find it helpful to learn a few things that will help you make your own mind up about the quality of a Web site and the information it provides. Exhibit 3.1. provides guidelines on evaluating a Web site.

1. *Source:* Who provides the Web site? This should be the main way to determine a site's reliability and quality. Since federal government Web sites, and those affiliated with a college or university, are often the most trusted source of information, look for a URL ending in .gov or .edu. Though a URL ending in .org identifies a not-for-profit organization (see Glossary), which people usually view as being unbiased, it's important that you don't automati-

cally accept ".org" to indicate reliability since there are some ".org" Web sites sponsored by people who want to sell you something.

2. *Content:* Where did the information come from? Is there any clinical or scientific evidence (usually based on clinical trials: see Glossary) to support statements in support of a view or position. Medical facts and figures should have references, such as citations to articles in medical journals (you could do a PubMed search to check). Personal testimonials, such as, "Since I started taking your product I have never felt better and at age ninety have run my first marathon," are not evidence.

3. *Disclosure:* The mission or purpose of the site should be clearly stated, it should be up-front about its purpose. Any reliable Web site should include a statement regarding the mission of the sponsoring organization. Also, when a Web site asks for user input or registration, the purpose and use of obtaining that information should be disclosed. Some health-related Web sites are already collecting personal health information to "tailor" content, and as sites begin to integrate health care services and information, confidentiality and privacy safeguards will become increasingly important.

4. *Links:* High-quality sites have links to other high-quality sites. The National Institutes of Health (NIH) is a high-quality site— "Mary's Herbal Magic Garden and Goat Farm" is not.

5. *Design:* Though not essential to the quality of information a reputable site will put some thought into its design so that users can easily navigate and find information.

6. *Interactivity:* There should be a feedback mechanism so you can offer comments, corrections, and criticisms, and raise questions about the information provided.

7. *Referral:* The Web site should encourage you to discuss the information with your health care provider. Be very suspicious of sites that do not!

8. *Date:* When was the Web site last updated? It's important that medical information be current, so Web sites should be reviewed and updated on a regular basis.

You might also find it useful to look for the logo of the Health on the Net Foundation's Code of Conduct (HONcode):

The blue and red HONcode logo is displayed on Web sites that voluntarily agree to abide by the Health On the Net Foundation's Code of Conduct for publishing quality health information on the Internet. The logo is more likely to be displayed on Web sites that contain accurate health information.

Parents and guardians might also want to check that sites are appropriate for children. Several sites have been developed specifically for the information needs of young people (see Chapter 7). Some health sites may also have a section especially for children, teenagers, or parents.

WEB SITES FOR EVALUATING WEB CONTENT

The following Web sites and documents provide more detailed information and valuable discussions about using evaluation criteria for Web content.

Health on the Web: Finding Reliable Information
<http://familydoctor.org/783.xml>

A patient-friendly guide from the American Academy of Family Physicians (AAFP).

Health On the Net Foundation (HON)
<http://www.hon.ch/>

This site includes a description of the Health on the Net Code of Conduct, as well as the MedHunt medical search engine.

Medical Products and the Internet: A Guide to Finding Reliable Information
<http://www.who.int/>

A clearly written document from the World Health Organization (WHO). Also includes valuable guidance on buying medical products online. The URL for this document is rather long, so you can find the document by going to the homepage then typing the words *internet* and *reliable* into the search engine box.

QUICK: Quality Information Checklist
<http://www.quick.org.uk/menu.htm>

My favorite! Though designed to help children ages five to seven evaluate the quality of health sites, it's a useful and fun tool for all ages and explains this topic in clear, easy-to-understand language.

WHAT'S IN THE BOTTLE?
UNDERSTANDING PRODUCT LABELS

We'll drink a, drink a, drink,
To Lydia Pink a, Pink a, Pink
The savior of the human ra-hay-hayce
She invented a medicinal compound
Whose effects God can only replace.

Drinking song (1890s)

Until the early twentieth century many Americans used "patent medicines." These "medicines" were unregulated mixtures, claiming to cure or prevent everything, including veneral disease, tuberculosis, and cancer. One of the most popular patent cures was Miss Lydia E. Pinkam's "Vegetable Compound," promoted as a cure for "painful Complaints and Weaknesses so common to our best female population." The compound was almost 20 percent alcohol, which probably contributed to its popularity. Other popular cures of the day contained opium ("to put baby to sleep!"), and more harmful compounds such as mercury and formaldehyde. Legal reforms of the patent medicine and drug industry eventually resulted in congress passing the Pure Drug and Food Act of 1906, which prevented manufactures from promoting patent medicines as either medicines or cures. This attempt to regulate the drug industry eventually resulted in the founding of the Food and Drug Administration (FDA) in 1927.

Although the federal government regulates herbs through the FDA, herbs are currently regulated as foods or "dietary supplements" rather than as drugs. In general, the laws about putting herbs on the market are less strict than the laws for drugs. Pharmaceutical drugs take many years of research to develop, and the FDA does not approve new drugs until there have been several phases of study to show that they not only work but that they are safe to use. See Exhibit 3.2 for an outline of the four phases of a clinical trial. Although drug manufacturers are required to prove that their products are safe before being marketed, herbal products manufacturers do not have to. It is up to the FDA to prove that herbs on the market are unsafe. This is why you'll see this disclaimer on the label of herbal products: "This product has not been evaluated by the Food and Drug Administration. This product is not intended to diagnose, treat, cure or prevent any disease."

EXHIBIT 3.2.
The Four Phases of a Clinical Trial

Phase 1	The drug, or treatment, is tried in humans for the first time. The goal is not to see if it works, but to find out the most effective dose and see if there are any side effects. The focus is on safety.
Phase 2	The drug, or treatment, is tested in patients using the dosage and protocol determined in Phase 1.
Phase 3	The drug, or treatment, is tested in a large group of people to confirm its effectiveness, check on side effects, compare its effectiveness to other drugs and treatments, and collect information that will allow it to be used safely.
Phase 4	Studies are carried out after the drug has been approved for marketing to collect information on its long-term use.

The legal standards for processing, harvesting, or packaging of mainstream drugs are not applied when herbs are manufactured. Some companies apply their own standards, but many do not. The regulation of herbal remedies in the United States has been slow because they are considered "natural," so there is considerable public opposition to any form of regulation. Manufacturers of these products are not subjected to the same FDA scrutiny as pharmaceutical companies, so consumers are not afforded the same protections.

Some herbal products do not always contain the ingredients listed on the labels and you can't always be sure that two bottles of the same herb contain the same dose of active ingredient. A 2004 study of St. John's wort products purchased from California health food stores showed huge differences in the amount of active ingredient present in different brands and some people buying the popular herbal medicine may be getting almost none at all.[1] The FDA is currently developing regulations for "good manufacturing practices" (GMPs), which will likely guarantee that what's in a dietary supplement is pure and the strength and potency of the supplement reflects what's stated on the label. GMPs set factory standards for such things as cleanliness, equipment sanitation, sampling and testing ingredients, controlling contamination, and expiration dating.

More and more herbs are being sold as "standardized extracts." These products contain a specific concentration of one or more "marker" compounds, which are the compounds considered to be mainly responsible for an herb's therapeutic effect. Standardization refers to the process of delivering a product with a specified minimum level of one or more of these marker compounds. This can help guarantee that herbal products have the same potency from batch to batch during the manufacturing process. Making a standardized extract means knowing which are the active ingredients, and unfortunately, there are only a few herbs for which this is known: these include St. John's wort, *Ginkgo biloba*, kava, and ginseng. Identifying top-quality herb brands can be tricky but there are a few things you can look for before you purchase. These are summarized in Exhibit 3.3.

EXHIBIT 3.3.
A Guide to Choosing Herbal Products

- Look for standardized extracts.
- Many leading brands employ good manufacturing practices (GMPs) and will state that on the label.
- An expiration date should indicate that the manufacturer has procedures in place to test the shelf life of its products.
- Reputable manufacturers will include a telephone number or a Web site address on the label so you can ask questions about the product.
- Check if the bottle contains something to preserve freshness, such as silica and antioxidant packets, or comes with special airtight seals and amber glass packaging to help protect the product from light.
- Look for the "USP Dietary Supplement Verified" seal on a label, indicating that the supplement has met certain manufacturing standards.
- Look for a certification mark from The Good Housekeeping Institute, a consumer products testing lab associated with *Good Housekeeping* magazine. A certification mark indicates the product to be safe and effective.
- Look for a NSF mark on the label. Manufacturers pay a fee to be tested by NSF and can use the NSF mark on labels if products pass for accuracy, lack of contamination, and good manufacturing practices.

WEB SITES FOR DECODING
HERBAL PRODUCT LABELS

The following Web sites provide sound advice on things to look out for when buying and using herbal products and what to look for on the label. They are also useful for finding information about issues that affect the sale and availability of herbal supplements in the United States.

ConsumerLab.com
<http://www.comsumerla.com>

Buying natural remedies can be an iffy proposition since they're subject to little federal regulation.ConsumerLab.com (CL) promotes itself as "a leading provider of consumer information and independent evaluations of products that affect health and nutrition." Manufacturers pay a testing fee and results are proprietary to the manufacturer. However, if a product "passes," it will appear in CL's Web site listing of the respective *Product Review* and is also eligible to carry the CL Seal of Approval. Funded by private investors rather than the supplements industry, CL purchases products for testing from a selection of the top-selling brands. It tests for identity and potency, but not effectiveness, e.g., Does the product contain what the label claims? Is it truly ginseng or ginkgo, or something else? The site includes a helpful encyclopedia of information on herbs and supplements. Unfortunately most of the information is available only to paid subscribers.

Food and Drug Administration (FDA)
<http://www.fda.gov/>

In the United States, herbal preparations are not classified as drugs but as "dietary supplements," and are currently covered by the Dietary Supplement and Health Education Act (DSHEA) of 1994. From the FDA's homepage select "Food" (to access the Center for Food Safety & Applied Nutrition), then from "Program Areas" choose "Dietary Supplements" to locate details on DSHEA and to view FDA information on reported adverse reactions and fraudulent claims.

Dietary Supplements (from the FDA)
<http://www.cfsan.fda.gov/~dms/supplmnt.html>

Everything you've always wanted to know about the regulation of herbs and other dietary supplements but were afraid to ask can be found on this site. A good site if you want more background information on the strange twilight world of the regulation of herbs in the United States.

National Center for Complementary and Alternative Medicine
   (NCCAM): Clinical Trials
<http://nccam.nih.gov/clinicaltrials>

Provides a good overview of the clinical trial process, with information on clinical trials of complementary and alternative medicine taking place throughout the United States and the world. Useful advice is given for those who may wish to take part in such trials.

NSF International: Consumers
<http://www.nsf.org/consumer/>

NSF International is a not-for-profit, nongovernmental organization involved in standards development, product certification, and education for public health and safety. This is a useful Web site for learning about dietary supplement/herb issues, with sound advice on things to look out for when buying and using herbal products and what to look for on the label.

USP Verification Program
<http://www.usp.org/USPVerified/>

The United States Pharmacopeia (USP) is the official public standards-setting authority for all prescription and over-the-counter medicines, dietary supplements, and other health care products manufactured and sold in the United States. USP sets standards for the quality of these products and works with health care providers to help them reach the standards. The USP-Verified mark on a dietary supplement label indicates high-quality supplements. This Web site provides a list of which companies participate in the USP-Verified program and a list of verified supplements, plus where they're available.

GENERAL HEALTH AND CAM WEB SITES

All beginnings are somewhat strange; but we must have patience, and little by little, we shall find things, which at first were obscure, becoming clearer.

St. Vincent de Paul

Useful information on herbs can be found on several of the most widely used health and medicine Web sites, though it's sometimes difficult to actually find information buried within a site and many simply provide links to the more specialized sites listed in later chapters of this book. However, they can be useful starting points for gathering information, so this chapter lists some of the most popular ones. Over the past few years a number of Web sites devoted entirely to alternative therapies have appeared and I would suggest you try these sites first.

Sites listed in this section are sometimes referred to as "metasites." Metasites are guides to other Web sites. Most metasites are organized by topic, and include hypertext ("clickable") links to the Web sites they list. There are both general metasites and subject-specific metasites. Yahoo! is an example of a general metasite. The National Center for Complementary and Alternative Medicine (NCCAM) Web site is a subject-specific metasite.

You may have noticed that the title of this chapter includes the world "CAM." This stands for complementary and alternative medicine. It's a sort of umbrella term to refer to all those therapies or procedures people think of as being "alternative medicine." When you start checking the Internet for herbal information you'll notice that sometimes it's included under the heading "alternative medicine," sometimes "complementary medicine" and sometimes "complementary and alternative medicine" (CAM). You'll also come across sites listed under the heading "holistic" or "integrative medicine." I prefer CAM to refer to all those therapies or procedures commonly referred to as "alternative medicine" and will use it as such in this book.

Good metasites use subject experts (such as physicians) to review Web sites, and include only those that meet rules such as those discussed previously. Look on the site itself for information about who selects the links. When you find a Web site that meets your needs, be sure to use your browser to bookmark it or add it to your "favorites."

If you want to do a bit of Internet surfing, the trick is to find a few good Web sites, such as the site for NCCAM (see Figure 3.2 later in this chapter), then look on their pages for lists of "related resources," "links," or similar terminology. Many of the related resources will list other related resources, and so on.

The Alternative Medicine Homepage
<www.pitt.edu/~cbw/altm.html>

The Alternative Medicine Homepage was created by Charles B. Wessel, at the Falk Library of the Health Sciences, University of Pittsburgh. This is one of the best-known and most exhaustive lists of CAM sites on the Internet. It's a well-annotated guide and jump station to Internet resources, mailing lists, newsgroups, and bibliographic databases.

InteliHealth
<http://www.intelihealth.com/>

InteliHealth is a joint venture of Aetna U.S. Healthcare and Johns Hopkins University and Health System, with participation by a large number of health care organizations and agencies, including Harvard Medical School. The site is extremely rich in content and is easily navigated. At the homepage select Complementary & Alternative Medicine under Healthy Lifestyles.

healthfinder®
<http://www.healthypeople.gov/healthfinder/>

The healthfinder site is the federal government's gateway to reliable health information resources that have been carefully selected by the U.S. Department of Health and Human Services (DHHS). Every resource listed includes a brief description and contact information for the organization that produces it. It's useful, but not one of the best metasites for CAM. Find information by typing keywords into the search box.

Richard and Hinda Rosenthal Center for Complementary and Alternative Medicine
<http://www.rosenthal.hs.columbia.edu/>

The Rosenthal center is part of the Columbia Presbyterian Medical Center in New York City. Created in 1993, it was one of the first centers at a major medical school established to deal specifically with research, education, and training in complementary and alternative medicine. The CAM Research and Information Resources section contains some of the best descriptions of valuable information resources in the field of alternative and complementary medicine.

MayoClinic.com
<http://www.mayoclinic.com/>

The Mayo Clinic's award-winning consumer Web site features easy-to-understand information on health and medical topics, all reviewed for accuracy by Mayo Clinic personnel. Content includes interactive resources and tools, information on specific diseases and disorders, management of particular chronic conditions, suggestions for healthy lifestyles, consumer drug information, specialists' answers to frequently asked questions about diseases, and health decision-making guides. Click on the Drugs and Supplements tab to access comprehensive information about herbs from Natural Standard, widely considered one of the most authoritative and reliable CAM sources providing impartial evidence-based information about herbs and supplements.

MedlinePlus
<http://www.nlm.nih.gov/medlineplus/herbalmedicine.html>

Developed by the National Library of Medicine (NLM), Medline Plus is a gold mine of health information. It provides extensive health information in both English and Spanish and is updated daily. The site features an "A to Z" guide of health topics including a section on Herbal Medicine. Click on the Español button to switch to Spanish-language materials (see Figure 3.1).

National Center for Complementary and Alternative Medicine (NCCAM)
<http://www.nccam.nih.gov>

One of the most important events affecting the way U.S. medicine deals with CAM was the founding of the Office of Alternative Medicine (OAM) in 1992, later renamed the National Center for Complementary and Alternative Medicine (NCCAM). Funded by the U.S. government, NCCAM's mission is to promote research into the effectiveness of CAM practices, develop an understanding of how they work, and provide the American public with reliable information about their safety and effectiveness.

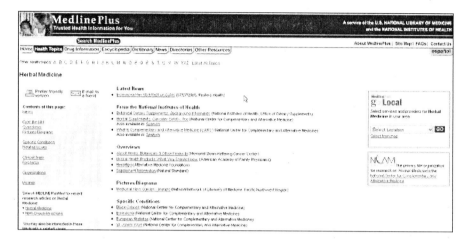

FIGURE 3.1. Medline Plus
<http://www.nlm.nih.gov/medlineplus/>

NCCAM supports and provides information for clinical trials involving herbal and other CAM therapies. A "clinical trial" is a research study to answer specific questions about new drugs, therapies, or new ways of using known treatments and is used to determine whether new drugs or new treatments are both safe and effective. New drugs are tested on people only after laboratory and animal studies show promising results. Clinical trials are conducted on CAM throughout the United States and the world. To find out more about clinical trials, and to find trials that are recruiting participants, go to the Clinical Trials section. You can search this site by the type of therapy being studied or by disease or condition (see Figure 3.2).

NOAH (New York Online Access to Health)
<http://www.noah-health.org/>

NOAH's mission is to provide accurate, timely, unbiased, and relevant consumer health information on a variety of health topics, in both English and Spanish. Go to Health Topics/Procedures and Medicine/Complementary and Alternative Therapies, then Herbal Medicine.

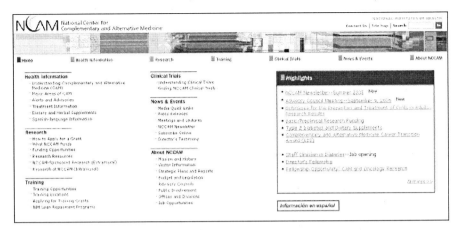

FIGURE 3.2. National Center for Complementary and Alternative Medicine (NCCAM)
<http://nccam.nih.gov/>

The Office of Dietary Supplements (ODS)
<http://ods.od.nih.gov>

In the United States, herbal preparations are not currently classified as drugs but instead are bundled into the food category "dietary supplements." The Office of Dietary Supplements (ODS), within the National Institutes of Health (NIH), supports research into all dietary supplements as well as promoting the dissemination of research results (see Figure 3.3). The ODS produces two very useful databases: the International Bibliographic Information on Dietary Supplements (IBIDS) and Computer Access to Research on Dietary Supplements (CARDS): IBIDS is discussed in Chapter 4.

WEIL™
<http://www.drweil.com/>

Andrew Weil, MD, is a Harvard-trained physician well-known for his promotion of alternative medical therapies within a conventional medical framework. Dr. Weil sponsors this site that contains a lot of information on complementary and alternative medicine. Unfortunately, there is a lack of scientific evidence to support many of his recommendations, and the site is now so commercial that it's difficult to tell what

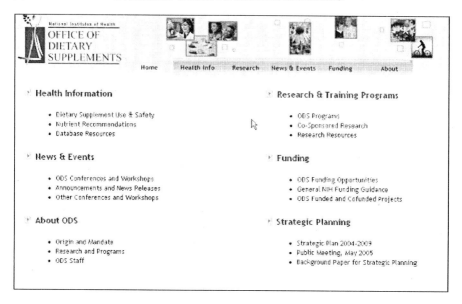

FIGURE 3.3. Homepage of the Office of Dietary Supplements (ODS)
<http://ods.od.nih.gov/>

is, and what is not, an advertisement—every page seems to have more
ads than useful information. That being said, it does contain much useful basic information on herbs. Its most useful feature is probably the
Ask Dr. Weil archives where Q&A on contemporary health issues
are submitted by readers with answers provided by Dr. Weil. Perhaps
the best way to navigate this site is to simply type search terms into the
search box on the homepage. However, make certain you check out
other Web sites for a second opinion.

NOTE

1. Wang, Zhao-Jun, Lin, Shih-Mei, and Hu, Miao-Lin. Contents of hypericin and
pseudohypericin in five commercial products of St John's wort *(Hypericum perforatum).
Journal of the Science of Food and Agriculture* 84(5): 395-397; April 15, 2004.

Chapter 4

Searching the Medical Literature

The beginning of wisdom is to call things by their right names.

Chinese Proverb

UNDERSTANDING THE SCIENCE OF HERBS

What exactly is an herb? Do I say "herb" or "erb?" Why do herbs have both a "common name" and "scientific name," and should I care? Are they different from botanicals? And why do people call them "dietary supplements?" If this isn't confusing enough, how am I supposed to pronounce words such as *Hypericum perforatum?* These and other terms are often used in the herbal literature, so you'll benefit from a basic understanding of why they're used and what they mean. This chapter will help you understand the words you'll frequently come across and point out some useful Web sites that you should visit for further information.

First, what exactly is an herb? For many people "herb" conjures up visions of soothing herbal teas such as chamomile or the bright green flakes of basil in spaghetti sauce. If you do any cooking you'll be familiar with common culinary herbs such as basil, mint, parsley, sage, etc. But what about the hawthorn tree, whose berries and flowers have been widely used for centuries to treat heart ailments? Then there's the bark from the slippery elm tree that's used to soothe sore throats. Are berries and bark "herbs?" Once you start browsing lists of medicinal herbs you'll come across many plants and plant parts that are rather different

Internet Guide to Herbal Remedies
© 2006 by The Haworth Press, Inc. All rights reserved.
doi:10.1300/5855_05

from the ones you use in the kitchen. To a botanist or a gardener, an herb is a plant that has no woody tissue and dies down to the ground at the end of a growing season—hence the gardening term "herbaceous border." However, today the word is used very loosely to refer to any plant part valued for its medicinal, savory, or aromatic qualities. As far as the pronunciation is concerned, both "herb" with an "h" and "erb" are correct but most Americans tend to drop the *h*.

Both print and online herbal resources usually list herbs by either their "scientific" or "common name." Understanding which is which, and why they're used, will help you navigate to the correct entry for a particular herb on many Web sites. Exhibit 4.1 lists various names used for the herb popularly known as St. John's wort. As you can see, several common names are often used in different regions or countries to refer to the same plant. To get around the problem of one plant having several different names, botanists give a plant one unique name, referred to as the scientific name (sometimes also referred to as the Latin or botanical name). Though a plant may have several different common names it will usually have only one scientific name. This is also sometimes re-ferred to as the Latin name since it's usually derived from the ancient Latin language, and consists of two parts (referred to as "binomial"): the first part indicates the genus (with capital first letter), which is a group of closely related plants, and the second part is specific for this

---

**EXHIBIT 4.1.
Names Used for St. John's Wort**

Common names   St. John's wort, Amber Touch-and-Heal,
                     Tipton Weed, Klamath Weed, John's Rosin Rose,
                     Johanniskraut (Germany),
                     Herb de millepertuis (France)

Latin name
Scientific name   } *Hypericum perforatum*
Botanical name

Pharmacopeial name: Hyperici herba

species (written entirely in lower case). Thus, *Echinacea purpurea,* or Eastern purple cornflower, refers to one species in the genus *Echinacea. Echinacea angustifolia,* though related, is an entirely different species. The scientific name is often abbreviated, as in *E. purpurea.* Technically, the full scientific name for an herb species also includes the name of the person who first described the species. Thus we have *Panax quinquefolius* L., for one species of "ginseng" first named by Swedish naturalist Linnaeus. Because Linnaeus named so many species, and is considered the "Father of Taxonomy," his name is usually abbreviated to just L. Many herbal resources list plants by both common and scientific names.

It often helps to remember scientific names if you know what the words actually mean. For example, echinacea is derived from the Greek "echinos," meaning hedgehog, and refers to the spiny seed heads. The scientific name for St. John's wort is *Hypericum perforatum. Perforatum* is Latin for "perforated," since the leaves show translucent dots when held up to the light, giving the impression that the leaf is perforated. The genus name *Hypericum* is thought to derive from two Greek words *hyper* and *eikon* for "over an icon," a reference to the practice of placing sprigs of the plant above images to clear the air of evil spirits. "Wort" is simply Old English for "plant."

Scientific names are usually derived from ancient Greek and Latin, but unfortunately there aren't any ancient Greeks or Romans around to tell us how to speak it. However, a general rule is to pronounce it as you would any English word but try to pronounce every syllable. Table 4.1 provides a pronunciation guide to several of the more popular scientific names.

Note in Exhibit 4.1 that there is also a third type of name you may come across: the pharmacopieal name. Not every part of a plant contains the active chemicals that make the herb effective. For example, St. John's wort is prepared from the plant's yellow flowers while ginseng is prepared from the roots and saw palmetto from the berries. Sometimes different parts of the same plant even yield different products. (The glossary at the end of this book includes definitions for some of the common plant terms you'll come across.) The pharmacopieal name is a convenient system for herbalists to identify an herbal preparation by referring both to a plant's scientific name and the plant part or type of preparation that is useful. Thus, a preparation made from the root of

TABLE 4.1. Guide to Pronouncing Scientific Names.

Common Name	Scientific Name	Pronunciation
Aloe	*Aloe vera*	AL-oh-e VE-ra
Black Cohosh	*Cimicifuga racemosa*	sim-iss-SIFF-yew-guh ra-sem-OH-suh
Chamomile	*Matricaria recutita*	mat-ri-KAR-ee-uh re-KOO-tee-ta
Chinese Ginseng	*Panax ginseng*	PAY-ax JIN-sing
Goldenseal	*Hydrastis canadensis*	hy-DRASS-tiss ka-na-DEN-sis
Evening Primrose	*Oenothera macrocarpa*	ee-NOTH-er-a ma-kro-KAR-pa
Garlic	*Allium sativum*	AL-lee-um sa-TEE-vum
Ginkgo	*Ginkgo biloba*	GINK-go bil-OW-buh
Purple Coneflower	*Echinacea purpurea*	ek-in AY-sha pur-PUR-ee-uh
Saw Palmetto	*Serona repens*	se-ROW-na REE-penz
St. John's wort	*Hypericum perforatum*	hye-PEHR-ik-um per-for-AY-tum
Valerian	*Valeriana officinalis*	val-err-ee-AY-nuh oh-fiss-ih-NAH-liss

echinacea is referred to as *Echinacea radix,* while one using the parts of the plant growing aboveground is known as *Echinacea herba.* Other common plant part names listed in herbal pharmacopeals are: bulbus, for bulb; cortex, for cortex or bark; flos, for flower; folium, for branch; semen, for seed; and spica, for flower spike.

When medicines are derived from herbs, they're often called phyto-medicines, botanicals, herbal products, or herbal supplements. To make matters a little more complicated, in the United States, herbal preparations are classified as "dietary supplements," along with vita-mins and minerals, and information on herbs is often listed under this term.

WEB SITES FOR BACKGROUND BOTANY

The following Web sites provide basic botanical information that will be useful in understanding herbal information you'll find on the

Internet. Some of the Web sites have photographs or drawings of the plants. Aside from their use in identification, some of these images are just strikingly beautiful.

BOTANY Online—The Internet Hypertextbook
<http://www.biologie.uni-hamburg.de/b-online/>

This is an online textbook on botany written by two professors at the University of Hamburg in Germany (but don't worry, the important parts are in English!). Includes brief chapters on the history of botany from ancient Egypt to present times and relevant sections such as how to identify plants, the parts of a plant, and important features of flowering plants.

Botany: Plant Parts and Functions
<http://ag.arizona.edu/pubs/garden/mg/botany/plantparts
.html>

This site is part of a manual compiled by the College of Agriculture at the University of Arizona and is an excellent introduction to basic botany. Chapter 1 includes useful information on the functions of stems, leaves, buds, roots, flowers, fruits, and seeds.

Dave's Garden
<http://davesgarden.com/>

Dave's Garden caters to the interests and needs of gardeners, farmers and horticulture professionals worldwide. The Plant Files section includes a useful guide to the pronunciation of the names of most herbs. Garden Terms is a useful glossary of plant and gardening terms.

The PLANTS Database
<http://plants.usda.gov/>

This is a project of the United States Department of Agriculture (USDA) and is a great resource for finding images of herbs and other plants (see Figure 4.1). Entries can be retrieved by both common and scientific names.

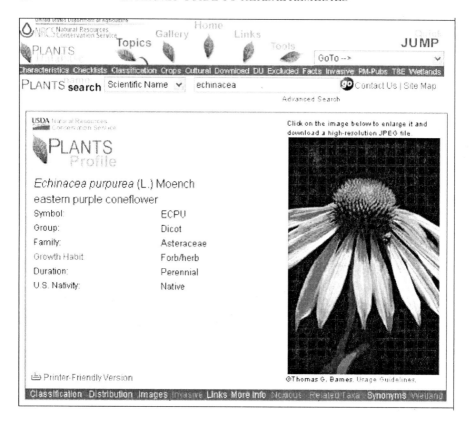

FIGURE 4.1. Echinacea Record from the USDA PLANTS Database
<http://plants.usda.gov/java/prfile?symbol=ECPU&photoID=ecpu_003_avp.tif>

THE IMPORTANCE OF MEDICAL JOURNALS

In 1984, Lorenzo Odone, a five-year-old boy living in Virginia was diagnosed with an incurable degenerative disease called adrenoleuko-dystrophy (ALD). ALD is a rare, inherited metabolic disorder. Symptoms include dementia, loss of sight, hearing, speech, and ability to walk, usually resulting in death within a couple of years. Frustrated by the medical profession's inability to help, his parents taught themselves biology and conducted an extensive search of the medical literature to develop a treatment for their son. Eventually they developed what came to be famously known as "Lorenzo's Oil" (Their story was immortalized in a film of the same name starring Nick Nolte and Susan Sarandon) .[1]

Back in 1984, before the days of free online access to the MEDLINE database, searching the medical literature was a difficult task. The Odones had to spend months in libraries, searching through the biomedical literature. However, with the advent of the Internet, and the National Library of Medicine (NLM)'s PubMed system this has now dramatically changed.

Many useful types of resources that health professionals use are available to consult, including books, journal articles, and Web sites. However, in medicine and the health sciences the most up-to-date reliable information is usually found in an article in a scholarly journal, published by and for experts. In order to be published in a scholarly journal, an article must first go through the peer-review process in which a group of widely acknowledged experts in a field reviews it for content, scholarly soundness, and academic value. The paper is the actual report of the work, and contains all of the details on the background, methods, results, and conclusions. In most cases, articles in scholarly journals present new, previously unpublished information.

To make the most of a database such as MEDLINE you should understand the difference between references, abstracts, and papers. References are just that: references to original published journal articles containing the title and author as well as the name of the journal, and the year, volume number, and page numbers. If you have a reference, you can look up the paper in a medical library. An abstract, however, is a short summary of the journal article and is something you can read to determine whether a paper is interesting enough to be worth a trip to the library. Almost all papers in MEDLINE and other high-quality medical databases contain abstracts for many of the references.

PUBMED (MEDLINE)

PubMed is the name of the system that provides free online access to MEDLINE, the foremost medical database in the world by using PubMed you can find citations and abstracts to articles in over 4,500 highly regarded medical journals. MEDLINE has been in use for more than thirty years—long before the Internet existed. Its content has saved lives, improved care, and provided answers to important questions posed by researchers and health care professionals. It is of great value to anyone looking for the latest medical research.

MEDLINE is usually the first step in investigating a new research area. The database is huge, containing information on over 15 million journal articles, so it's sometimes a little tricky to find the information you want. To make searching easier, government-funded agencies such as the National Center for Complementary and Alternative Medicine (NCCAM) and the Office of Dietary Supplements (ODS) have created free online databases for members of the public to search for the latest journal articles. The two most useful ones are "CAM on PubMed" and the International Bibliographic Information on Dietary Supplements (IBIDS) database (pronounced E-bids).

GOOGLE VERSUS PUBMED

Why use PubMed and not Google? First, Google emphasizes Web sites that are popular, as measured by the number of links from other sites, and does not give much weight to quality. You'll be frustrated by the large number of links Google will generate for common topics and the best information is often buried in the search results. Second, there's a lot of junk in Google searches. Unlike Google and other Internet search engines, MEDLINE is selective in what it indexes and the information comes from high-quality, peer-reviewed journals. Third, PubMed has powerful search features designed to help you zero in on the most important articles.

You can also use the Internet to access more specialized databases, providing more detailed information on herbs, such as the names of the active chemical in herbal preparations and the uses of medicinal plants by traditional healing systems. The Rosenthal Center Directory of Databases provides information about and links to these sources.

WEB SITES FOR LINKS TO DATABASES, TECHNICAL INFORMATION, AND PUBLISHED RESEARCH

The following sites provide information and links to databases for those interested in finding more in-depth or up-to-date information on herbs. Much of this information is a little technical, and primarily aimed at the health professional, but resources such as the IBIDS database will allow you to find newsletters, newspaper articles, and other consumer publications written in easily understandable language.

MEDLINE (Pubmed)
<http://www.ncbi.nlm.nih.gov/PubMed/>

MEDLINE includes the journal literature of medicine, nursing, dentistry, veterinary medicine, the health care system, and the preclinical sciences such as anatomy and biochemistry. It currently contains references to around 15 million articles, from over 4,500 journals, now dating back to the 1950s. Around 33,000 new citations are added each month! However, not every journal is indexed from cover to cover and some are "selectively indexed:" if an article is not related to biomedicine it is not added to MEDLINE. Since June 1997 MEDLINE has been available free on the Internet through the PubMed site. PubMed is a World Wide Web (www) retrieval service developed by the National Center for Biotechnology Information (NCBI) at the National Library of Medicine (NLM). Updated daily, PubMed provides a free search interface for the MEDLINE database.

All records in the MEDLINE database consist of two parts: a bibliographic citation and a list of indexing terms (see Exhibit 4.2). The bibliographic citation contains everything you need to know to locate the original article: title, author(s), and journal information. However, the citations themselves often do not contain enough information to allow you to easily find them in a database as large as MEDLINE. To add more information to a citation, professional indexers at the NLM add indexing terms to the Subject Field of the MEDLINE record from a standardized list of medical terms called Medical Subject Headings (MeSH).

EXHIBIT 4.2.
A MEDLINE Citation

Mycoses. 2004 Apr;47(3-4):87-92

Herbal medicines for treatment of fungal infections: A systematic review of controlled clinical trials.

Martin KW, Ernst E.

Complementary Medicine, Peninsula Medical School, Universities of Exeter and Plymouth, Exeter, UK.

Traditional medicine has made use of many different plant extracts for treatment of fungal infections and some of these have been tested for in vitro antifungal activity. This systematic review evaluates antifungal herbal preparations that have been tested in controlled clinical trials. Four electronic databases were searched for controlled clinical trials of antifungal herbal medicines. *(Abstract truncated).*

MeSH Terms:

- Antifungal Agents/therapeutic use
- Controlled Clinical Trials
- Humans
- Mycoses/drug therapy
- Phytotherapy
- Plant Extracts/therapeutic use
- Plants, Medicinal/chemistry
- Tea Tree Oil/therapeutic use
- Tinea/drug therapy

PubMed has become a major resource for up-to-date, current research in complementary and alternative medicine (CAM). Unfortunately, locating research on herbs can sometimes be tricky. One major problem is the confusion surrounding which names to use as search terms. For example, an article discussing milk thistle may refer to its common name (milk thistle), or its scientific name *(Silybum marianum),* or simply to one of its bioactive chemical constituents (e.g., silymarin). For the most commonly used herbs you can just type in the common name.

For an introduction to searching PubMed go to the PubMed home-page and click on Tutorial in the blue column. This site has extensive help on using the database. For a more detailed description of searching for herbal and other CAM information in PubMed see the handout writ-ten by library staff at Bastyr University (URL listed in this chapter) or the paper by Saxton and Owen.[2]

How do you get the complete journal article itself? The PubMed sys-tem provides something called LinkOut, which is a list of PubMed journals that provide links to full-text articles. Links are supplied by full-text providers, and though some articles are free many journals usually require registration, a subscription fee, or some other type of fee to access the full text. Switch to the Abstract display to see if a pub-lisher's icon link to the full text or select the LinkOut display from the Display menu. If the text is not available online, LinkOut provides a list of libraries that subscribe to the journal. Your local public or medical li-brary may also subscribe to the journal or give you advice on getting the article.

Bastyr University: Complementary and Alternative Medicine (CAM) Research Using MEDLINE
<http://www.bastyr.edu/library/resources/researchguide/ cammedline.asp>

The library staff at Bastyr University, a leading naturopathic college, have written a superb online guide to searching MEDLINE for CAM research.

CAM on PubMed
<http://www.nlm.nih.gov/nccam/camonpubmed.html>

CAM on PubMed is a joint venture of the National Center for Com-plementary and Alternative Medicine (NCCAM) and the National Library of Medicine (NLM). The database provides journal citations related to complementary and alternative medicine (CAM) and is in-tended for use by health professionals, CAM practitioners, researchers, educators, and consumers. It is essentially a subset of the MEDLINE database. Though the experienced searcher can probably get the same results using the parent PubMed database, this smaller database is obviously easier to deal with. Search it the same way as you would PubMed.

Combined Health Information Database (CHID)
<http://chid.nih.gov/>

CHID is a bibliographic database produced by health-related agencies of the federal government, including the Centers for Disease Control (CDC), the Office of Disease Prevention and Health Promotion, the Department of Veterans Affairs, and the National Center for Complementary and Alternative Medicine (NCCAM). The database provides bibliographic citations for major health journals, books, reports, pamphlets, audiovisuals, hard-to-find information resources, and health education/promotion programs. Go to Detailed Search, and under Select A Database for Searching, select Complementary and Alternative Medicine (CAM).

HerbMed®
<http://www.herbmed.org>

HerbMed is a database providing links to the scientific evidence from MEDLINE and other resources on the use of medicinal herbs. It is an unbiased, evidence-based information resource provided by the nonprofit Alternative Medicine Foundation. For each herb, you can find out clinical data, traditional uses, warnings, etc. For example, look at the adverse and toxic effects of echinacea and you'll get a brief description and links to the relevant report in PubMed where you can read the abstract.

Google Scholar®
<www.google.com>

Google has launched a new service called Google Scholar (select Scholar from the Google homepage) that searches for scholarly materials such as peer-reviewed (see glossary) journal articles, theses, books, and technical reports. Some information is available as full text, though in some instances only abstracts are displayed with links to pay document delivery services. Google Scholar is still in development and has serious limitations. It does not compare with PubMed for finding the most up-to-date health information. Be careful—it includes some MEDLINE citations but not the most recent ones. You should use PubMed MEDLINE for finding the most current peer-reviewed clinical information and medical research. However, it's a useful research tool and in some ways complements PubMed.

International Bibliographic Information on Dietary Supplements (IBIDS) Database
<http://ods.od.nih.gov/databases/ibids.html>

The International Bibliographic Information on Dietary Supplements (IBIDS) database (pronounced E-bids) is produced by the Office of Dietary Supplements (ODS) and the U.S. Department of Agriculture, and is designed to provide ready access to the international scientific literature on vitamins, minerals, hormonal products, and botanicals (see Figure 4.2). You can select from the IBIDS Consumer Database,

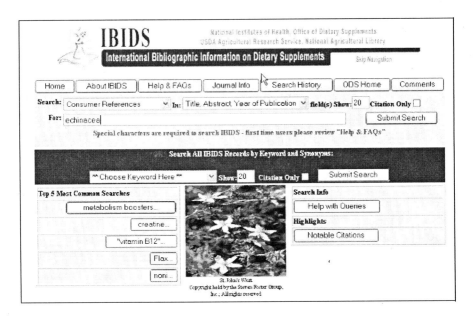

FIGURE 4.2. The IBIDS Database
<http://grande.nal.usda.gov/ivids/>

the Full IBIDS Database, or Peer Reviewed Citations Only. Peer-reviewed journals have a board of experts or "peers" who evaluate articles submitted for publication. The IBIDS Consumer Database restricts searches to references that have been selected from journals which provide dietary supplement information geared specifically toward consumers, rather than scientists.

Rosenthal Center: Directory of Databases
<http://www.rosenthal.hs.columbia.edu/Databases.html>

The Richard and Hinda Rosenthal Center is part of Columbia Presbyterian Medical Center in New York, and is one of the first centers at a major medical school devoted specifically to research, education, and training in complementary and alternative medicine. This Web page has a detailed list of databases available in the United States, Europe, and Asia, and is designed to facilitate research by both professionals and the public. It includes information on major biomedical bibliographic databases other than PubMed (e.g., EMBASE), major databases specific to complementary and alternative medicine (e.g., Allied and Complementary Medicine Database [AMED]), important pharmaceutical databases relevant to herbal medicine (e.g., NAtural PRoducts ALERT [NAPRALERT]), and traditional medicine databases (e.g., American Indian Ethnobotany Database, and Dr. Duke's Phytochemical and Ethnobotanical Databases which covers ethnobotanical uses for plants).

University of Washington Medicinal Herb Garden
<http://nnlm.gov/pnr/uwmhg/>

This site is designed to be a hypertext tour of the University of Washington's Medicinal Herb Garden. The actual 2.5-acre garden is the largest of its kind in the United States and was designed to serve as a source of information about the uses of herbaceous plants in traditional medicine and in the home and garden. This Web site is a sort of one-stop resource for information on herbs, including images and links to PubMed and more specialized databases. Be aware, though, it is only a "partial catalog," but you'll find entries for common herbs such as St. John's wort and echinacea. To retrieve journal citations go to the entry for an herb and click on "MEDLINE Citations vis PubMed." Also includes links to databases such as the full text of *Modern Herbal,* an exhaustive resource containing information on over 800 varieties of medicinal, culinary, and cosmetic herbs. If you use *Mrs. Grieve's* please note that it was written over seventy years ago, and there is little scientific evidence to support many of the recommendations.

NOTES

1. Maslin, J. Lorenzo's Oil: Parents Fighting to Keep Their Child Alive, *New York Times.* December 30, 1992; p. C7.

2. Saxton JD, and Owen DJ. Developing Optimal Search Strategies for Finding Information on Herbs and Other Medicinal Plants in MEDLINE. *J Altern Complement Med* 1(4):725-731, 2005.

Chapter 5

Herbal Safety and Efficacy

Sure, everyone always said, "Socrates, what is the meaning of life?" Or, "Socrates, how can I find happiness?" Did anyone ever say "Socrates, hemlock is poison"?*

Source unknown

ARE HERBS SAFE?

Let me begin this chapter by stating that the majority of herbs widely sold and distributed in the United States and Europe as capsules, tablets, and teas are safe. When herbs are used correctly, they are as safe as conventional medications, and often have fewer side effects. That being said, you should be aware that there are some very hazardous herbs currently on the market and others which may be harmful if not used correctly.

First, remember that just because something is touted as being "natural" doesn't necessarily mean that it's safe and won't harm you. Mushrooms may be "natural," and, in general, you won't come to any harm from eating those you buy at your local grocery store. However, some species such as the death cap *(Amanita phalloides)* can be deadly and people routinely die after mistakenly picking and eating the wrong kind

---

*Socrates was a famous Greek philosopher. He was forced to commit suicide by drinking a cup of hemlock. Hemlock *(Conium maculatum)* is found in Europe and parts of Asia and North America, and is a poisonous herb that looks a great deal like parsley.

Internet Guide to Herbal Remedies
© 2006 by The Haworth Press, Inc. All rights reserved.
doi:10.1300/5855_06

of mushroom. Some herbs contain powerful substances, which can have harmful effects if used in too high a dose or over long periods of time. Even some widely used herbs may have harmful effects if not used correctly. For example, it is possible for anyone to have an allergic reaction to just about anything and some people develop allergic reactions to chamomile and other herbs. Some evidence suggests that some commonly used herbs may cause undesirable effects during surgery. The American Society of Anesthesiologists (ASA) recommends that all herbal medications be discontinued two to three weeks before an operation (see entry in this chapter for ASA).

No drug is completely harmless, whether it's ginkgo extract or aspirin. Many medications, including herbals, have powerful ingredients that interact with the human body in different ways. The foods we eat, our lifestyle, and illness can all have an impact on our body's reaction to any drugs or herbs we ingest. Many people develop what are known as adverse drug reactions (ADRs). These unwanted reactions can be of two kinds. A "side effect" is usually something expected and mild: for example, if you take an antihistamine to control allergy symptoms drowsiness is considered an annoying, unwanted side effect. Most people only experience mild side effects and find them easily manageable. Adverse effects are unexpected, and can be more serious. You should always check to see if there are any known adverse effects associated with a certain herb.

Many patients, probably because they view all herbs as harmless, often don't see any need to tell their doctor that they're using herbs. Wrong! Health professionals are becoming increasingly concerned about the risk of interactions between herbs and prescription drugs. Some herbal medicines may cancel the effect of a prescription drug, others may reduce it, or even exaggerate it. St. John's wort, for example, interacts with AIDS drugs, chemotherapy, and birth control pills, making them less effective.[1] Herb-drug interactions often can't be predicted, so it's best to play it safe: do some research and tell your doctor.

You should be particularly careful when shopping for herbal medicines, since there are few standards that regulate how they're manufactured, and they receive little attention once they are on the market. Unlike conventional drugs, they are not tested and approved for safety or effectiveness by the Food and Drug Administartion (FDA) and can be removed from the market only after they've been shown to be harmful.

Furthermore, there are almost no standards that regulate how herbal products are manufactured, so sometimes you may never really know what you're really getting. You must be particularly careful using, for example, Chinese herbs, since there are reports of preparations being contaminated with poisonous minerals such as lead and mercury.[2]

I hope the preceding paragraphs have not sent you rushing to your medicine cabinet to throw all your herbal medicines in the garbage. As I stated at the beginning of this chapter, the vast majority of herbal products sold in the United States are safe, and in general seem to be less harmful than many conventional drugs. Just don't start taking them without doing a little research. Be especially careful if there's any chance they may interact with other medications you're taking. Perhaps most important of all, discuss the information with your doctor.

WEB SITES THAT DISCUSS HERBAL SIDE EFFECTS AND HERB/DRUG INTERACTIONS

Thankfully, reliable information on real or possible adverse effects associated with many herbs is now widely available. Most of the following sites also provide information on herb/drug interactions.

American Society of Anesthesiologists (ASA):
Patient Education Website
<http://www.asahq.org/patientEducation.htm>

Some evidence suggests that herbal remedies may cause complications during an operation. The ASA provides a patient education brochure, *What You Should Know About Herbal Use and Anesthesia,* that you can print out.

Familydoctor.org
<http://familydoctor.org/>

This site is sponsored by the American Academy of Family Physicians (AAFP), one of the largest national medical organizations. All of the information on this site has been written and reviewed by physicians and patient-education professionals at the AAFP. It provides easy-to-understand information for patients and the general public, including herbal and alternative remedies. Unfortunately, it includes comprehensive information for only the most widely used herbs such as echinacea. For example, you'll find information about ginger in the section on treatments for nausea. Type the name of the herb in the search box to find information.

GNCLiveWell
<http://www.gnc.com>

General Nutrition Centers (GNC) is a major national chain specializing in herbs and supplements. The Web site provides access to Healthnotes, a resource providing up-to-date information on all CAM therapies. Healthnotes is written by licensed medical professionals and provides descriptions for over 350 herbal remedies, indexed by common and scientific (botanical) name, including Western, Chinese, and Ayurvedic herbs. Articles also provide dosage and safety information. Ignore all the ads and go straight to the Herbal Remedies index under Healthnotes.

Consumer Advice on Food Safety, Nutrition and Cosmetics
University of Maryland Medical Center: Interactions
by Herb or Supplement
<http://www.umm.edu/altmed/ConsLookups/InteractionsBy
HerbSupp.html>

This site was created by the Center for Integrative Medicine (CIM), an interdepartmental center within the University of Maryland School of Medicine. It contains easy-to-read articles about herbs, including how they are used and how to take them. Additional information includes precautions and possible interactions, and a listing of associated research. Useful information is provided about interactions between specific drugs and herbal supplements (see Figure 5.1).

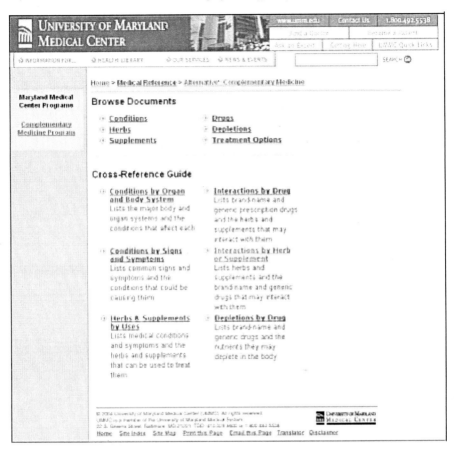

FIGURE 5.1. University of Maryland Medical Center: Herb and Drug Interactions <http://www.umm.edu/altmed/ConsLookups/InteractionsByHerbSupp.html> Reprinted with permission.

Ephedra Guide
<http://www.umm.edu/features/ephedra.html>

The herbal supplement ephedra has been the subject of controversy for some time. In 2003 the U.S. Food and Drug Administration announced a ban on dietary supplements containing ephedra because of associated health risks such as heart attacks and stroke. This guide from the University of Maryland Medical Center provides useful information and advice.

Mayoclinic.com: Natural Standard
<http://www.mayoclinic.com/>

The Drugs and Supplements section on the Mayoclinic.com Web site provides access to fact sheets compiled by Natural Standard, an international research collaboration that provides high-quality information on complementary and alternative medical therapies. Natural Standard analyzes thousands of scientific studies to provide in-depth information about effectiveness, safety, interactions, and use during pregnancy and breast-feeding. The focus is on the therapeutic "bottom line" of treatment safety and effectiveness. The evidence indicating whether a therapy/herb might really work is graded from A (strong scientific evidence that it works) to F (it likely does not work).

Memorial Sloan-Kettering Cancer Center:
About Herbs, Botanicals and Other Products
<http://www.mskcc.org/mskcc/html/11570.cfm>

The Memorial Sloan-Kettering Cancer Center (MSKCC) is one of the world's oldest and largest private institutions at the forefront of scientific research into cancer treatments, as well as the development of innovative cancer therapies and new patient care programs. Though primarily aimed at the cancer patient, the Herbs and Botanicals section provides useful information on which herbs may pose a health risk if taken incorrectly, which ones are likely to contain contaminants, which might cause dangerous interactions or increase bleeding, and which ones may cause photosensitivity and should not be used when undergoing radiation therapy.

Office of Dietary Supplements (ODS):
Health Information
<http://dietary-supplements.info.nih.gov/>

The Office of Dietary Supplements (ODS) was established to promote knowledge and understanding of dietary supplements by evaluating scientific information, stimulating and supporting research, dis-seminating research results, and to educate the public. Information includes Botanical Supplement Fact Sheets and a section on Consumer Safety.

Longwood Herbal Taskforce (LHTF)
<http://www.longwoodherbal.org/>

Highly recommended! The LHTF is a collaboration between faculty, staff, and students from Children's Hospital, the Massachusetts College of Pharmacy and Health Sciences, and the Dana Farber Cancer Institute. This site provides reviews of current literature on selected herbal supplements, including in-depth monographs, clinician information summary, and, for some herbs, a patient fact sheet you can print out.

University of Maryland Medical Center Complementary
Medicine Program
<http://www.umm.edu/altmed/index.html>

This online medical library provides an excellent guide to the use of individual herbs, with a special section on herbal supplements and the brand-name and generic drugs that may interact with them.

LET THE BUYER BEWARE:
FRAUD AND QUACKERY

"Bust enhancing" or "breast enlargement" supplements are now widely marketed to young women. These products contain various combinations of herbs, the most popular being hops, saw palmetto, damiana *(Turnera diffusa),* dong quai, chaste tree berry, blessed thistle, dandelion, wild yam *(Dioscorea villosa),* kava, fennel, black cohosh, and fenugreek. Ads regularly appear on television, on the Internet, and in magazines, and claim to offer a nonsurgical "natural" way to increase breast size and firmness. Unfortunately, no clinical trials have been carried out to test whether these herbs work. Instead, they usually rely on personal testimonials. An edition of the television program 20/20 even claimed that the people providing these testimonials are often paid actors, and the differences shown in "before and after" pictures are most likely the results of push-up bras.

Though fraud and quackery can occur throughout medicine, they tend to thrive in areas that do not have much scientific support or where the medical establishment is mistrusted. With more and more consumers using the Internet to find health information, the opportunities for fraud have significantly increased. Those who promote health fraud are being intentionally deceiving, and they know that their product doesn't do what they say it does. In contrast, quackery involves people who really believe their system or therapy works. Unfortunately, exotic, unproven, or exaggerated claims for herbs and other CAM therapies are widespread and sometimes even a physician has difficulty separating the serious science from the quackery.

As usual, I don't mean to scare you. Just keep your wits about you if you come across an unusual herbal remedy that interests you. Remember that if something sounds too good to be true, it usually is! Avoid anything that talks about "anti-aging" treatments, promises "quick and easy cures," or contains words such as "miraculous," "exclusive," "magic," or "secret."

The Federal Trade Commission (FTC) is responsible for monitoring the advertising of herbs and other supplements, in print and broadcast advertisements, infomercials, catalogs, and similar direct-marketing materials. Such advertising must be truthful and not misleading. The FTC has taken action against supplement manufacturers, advertising agencies, distributors, retailers, catalog companies, and others involved in the deceptive promotion of herbal products. The FTC's "Health Claims on the Internet" document has valuable advice on how to spot health fraud. Other Web sites listed are for organizations set up to protect the consumer from fraud and quackery and provide valuable advice for anyone using the Internet for health information or buying health products.

If you regularly use the Internet for health information you might want to browse these sites to help identify any fraudulent claims you may come across.

WEB SITES DEDICATED TO CONSUMER AWARENESS

Health Claims on the Internet: Buyer Beware (FTC)
<http://www.ftc.gov/bcp/conline/features/healthclaims.htm>

The Federal Trade Commission (FTC) works to prevent fraudulent, deceptive, and unfair business practices in the marketplace and to provide information to help consumers spot, stop, and avoid them. This document has valuable information on how to spot fraudulent claims for herbs and other supplements on the Internet.

American Council on Science and Health (ACSH)
<http://www.acsh.org/>

The American Council on Science and Health, Inc. (ACSH) is a nonprofit dedicated to the education of consumers on issues relating to food, nutrition, chemicals, pharmaceuticals, lifestyle, the environment, and health.

Center for Science in the Public Interest (CSPI)
<http://www.cspinet.org/>

The CSPI was founded in 1971 by scientists who had previously worked for Ralph Nader's Center for the Study of Responsive Law. The center is a nonprofit education and advocacy organization that focuses on improving the safety and nutritional quality of the food supply. Use the search engine box to locate articles from the Supplement Watch section.

ConsumerLab.com
<http://www.consumerlab.com>

ConsumerLab.com is an independent research laboratory that investigates the product quality of commercially available dietary supplements, including herbal products. ConsumerLab.com aims to test natural products to see if they meet scientific standards for potency, purity and consistency. You must pay for the complete reports but summaries are free (see Figure 5.2).

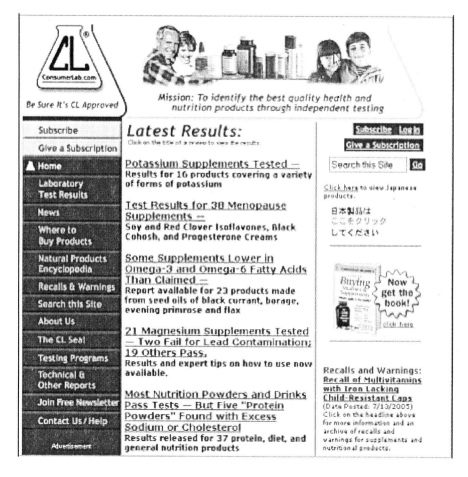

FIGURE 5.2. Homepage of ConsumerLab.com
<http://www.consumerlab.com>
Reprinted with permission.

Consumer Reports
<http://www.consumerreports.org/>

Consumer Reports is published by Consumers Union, a nonprofit organization known for publishing accurate reviews and comparisons of consumer products based on results from its in-house testing laboratory. Use the Site Map to go the Drugs and Supplements section. A subscription is required to view many of the reports.

**Tips for the Savvy Supplement User: Making
Informed Decisions
<http://www.fda.gov/fdac/features/2002/202_supp.htm.>**

This site has tips from the FDA to to help consumers become savvy dietary supplement users. Includes useful information about what to look out for when buying herbal products.

NOTES

1. Izzo AA. Drug interactions with St. John's Wort (Hypericum perforatum): A reveiw of the clinical evidence. *Int J Clin Pharmacol Ther* 42(3):139-148; 2004.
2. Ernst E. Toxic heavy metals and undeclared drugs in Asian herbal medicines. *Trends Pharmacol Sci* 23(3):136-139; 2002.

Chapter 6

Diseases and Conditions

There are no non-healing herbs—only the lack of knowledge.

Avicenna

Herbs and herbal therapies are available for almost every disease and health condition, and from a wide variety of healing systems. According to the World Health Organization (WHO), 80 percent of the world's population uses herbal remedies for some aspect of health care. In many developing countries, traditional medicine is still the main source of primary health care and medicinal herbs play a major role ("traditional medicine" refers to systems of healing that are not based on the Western scientific approach). China and the Indian subcontinent have developed the two most widely known systems, referred to respectively as Traditional Chinese Medicine (TCM) and Ayurvedic medicine. In both of these healing systems, herbs have a significant role and are increasingly gaining attention from Western medicine.

Herbs are currently being investigated to treat anxiety, arthritis, depression, high blood pressure, hormonal imbalances such as premenstrual tension, insomnia, migraines, nausea, poor blood circulation, and skin problems such as eczema. This section provides Web sites that contain information on herbs used for common health problems. Some of these herbs are widely known, and there is a respectable amount of information available on their use, while others are only now being investigated but show great promise.

Internet Guide to Herbal Remedies
© 2006 by The Haworth Press, Inc. All rights reserved.
doi:10.1300/5855_07

AIDS/HIV AND SEXUALLY TRANSMITTED DISEASES (STDs)

Sexually transmitted diseases (STDs) (such as hepatitis B and genital herpes) and acquired immunodeficiency syndrome (AIDS) have gained importance due to rapid spread of the diseases, the high cost of treatment, and the increased risk of transmission of other STDs. Current therapies available for treatment of STDs and AIDS are quite expensive and are associated with the emergence of drug resistance. Many patients with STDs and AIDS are therefore seeking help from alternative medicines such as Chinese and Ayurvedic medicine.

Several plant extracts have now been shown to inhibit the replication of the HIV virus, including plants from Panama, Indonesia, and those found in Ayurvedic medicine. A South African plant, *Sutherlandia frutescens,* the so-called "cancer bush," is gaining international attention as a potential inexpensive immune booster in the treatment of HIV/AIDS. There is also preliminary evidence that it has anti-HIV activity.[1]

Bulletin of Experimental Treatments for AIDS (BETA)
<http://www.sfaf.org/beta/>

BETA is published quarterly (in winter, spring, summer, and fall) by the Treatment and Education Center of the San Francisco AIDS Foundation (SFAF). It covers new developments in AIDS treatment research with in-depth articles on current treatments for HIV-positive individuals and AIDS-related illnesses. At the homepage select Browse by Topic, then Alternative/Complementary Treatments.

ALZHEIMER'S DISEASE/DEMENTIA

Alzheimer's disease (AD) is a progressive, degenerative brain disease that attacks the brain and results in problems such as memory loss, impaired thinking, agitation, and anxiety. It is the most common cause of dementia in the elderly and affects at least 3 to 4 million people in the United States. Over the years, several herbs have reportedly been useful in improving memory in old age: ginkgo, hawthorn berries, ginseng, sage *(Salvia officinalis),* and lemon balm *(Melissa officinalis)* are the five most commonly mentioned. Several studies show the significant benefits of aromatherapy on reducing agitation in patients with advanced Alzheimer's, particularly lavender and lemon oil (see the section on Depression for more information on aromatherapy).

University of Maryland Medical Center: Herbs and Supplements for Alzheimers
<http://www.umm.edu/altmed/ConsLookups/ Uses/Alzheimersdisease.html>

A superb site with information on herbs and other supplements for Alzheimer's disease, including comprehensive reviews of ginkgo, American ginseng, cat's claw *(Uncaria tomentosa),* and lemon balm (see Figure 6.1).

ANXIETY

Anxiety is difficult to describe. It affects how we feel, how we behave and has very real physical symptoms that can sometimes be mistaken for physical illness. Mild anxiety is vague and unsettling: severe anxiety can be extremely debilitating. Kava has been approved in Germany for anxiety as an over-the-counter medication since 1990 and in the United States is the ninth best-selling herb. Studies show a significant reduction of anxiety in patients taking kava extract.

University of Maryland Medical Center
<http://www.umm.edu/altmed/ConsConditions/ Anxietycc.html>

Comprehensive information about the signs and symptoms of anxiety and links to fact sheets on kava kava, lavender, lemon balm, passion flower, skullcap, and St. John's wort.

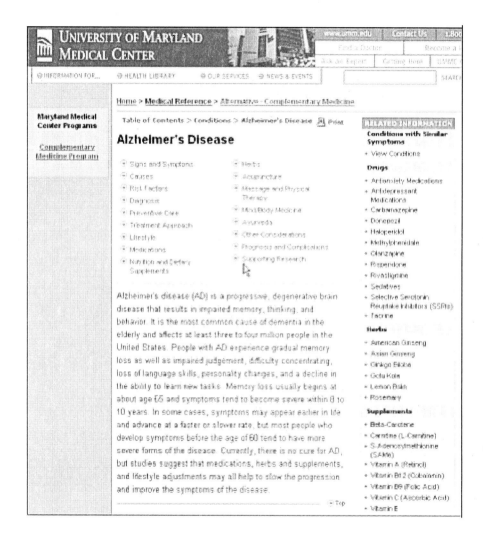

FIGURE 6.1. University of Maryland Medical Center: Herbs and Supplments for Alzheimer's Disease
<http://www.umm.edu/altmed/ConsLookups/Uses/Alzheimers disease.html>
Reprinted with permission.

ARTHRITIS

Osteoarthritis is a type of arthritis that is caused by the breakdown and eventual loss of cartilage in the joints. Several herbs show great promise in treating this condition: ginger is being studied for the treatment of osteoarthritis of the knee, and capsaicin cream (capsaicin is an ingredient found in cayenne peppers) is a safe and effective treatment for relieving pain.

Rheumatoid arthritis is an autoimmune disease that causes chronic inflammation of the joints. Autoimmune diseases occur when the body is mistakenly attacked by its own immune system. Cat's claw is a common name for at least twenty plants with sharp, curved thorns native to Central and South American tropical rain forests. Two of them, *Uncaria tomentosa* (UT) and *Uncaria guianensis* (UG) have a history of use in the treatment of rheumatoid arthritis.

The Arthritis Foundation
<http://www.arthritis.org/>

The Arthritis Foundation Web site has a section devoted entirely to supplements, including herbs such as black current oil *(Ribes nigrum),* cat's claw, devil's claw *(Harpagophytum procumbens),* and Thunder God Vine *(Tripterygium wilfordii).*

CANCER

We cannot change the direction of the wind, but we can adjust our sails.

Source unknown

The Internet is frequently used by cancer patients wishing to find information about their cancer and its treatment. Some patients want to know more about complementary and alternative medicine (CAM), especially if conventional cancer treatments don't seem to be effective or are difficult to endure and have severe side effects. About one-third of people with cancer have tried one or more CAM treatments, with dietary and herbal treatments being used by about 30 percent of cancer patients.[2] Many cancer patients don't expect CAM treatments to cure their cancer but use them to treat pain or control the side effects of chemotherapy. Ginger *(Zingiber officinale)*, for example, is beneficial for reducing the nausea and vomiting associated with chemotherapy.[3]

Growing evidence suggests that many plant compounds may be useful in the prevention of cancer and new approaches to cancer treatment now recognize the importance of diet and the protective effect of compounds found in herbs and other plants. Studies have shown that people in Southeast Asian countries have far lower risks of developing most cancers compared with those in North America, and it is thought that the consumption of certain vegetables and foods containing garlic, ginger, cayenne, turmeric, and soy play a key role. Several studies support the use of green tea *(Camellia sinensis)* in the prevention and treatment of various forms of cancer.[4] A significant body of evidence shows the positive role of herbs in combination with conventional cancer treatments. In studies with mice, *Ginkgo biloba* extract enhanced the radiation effect on tumors without increasing damage to normal tissue.[5] Grape seed extract (GSE) has shown similar results in the treatment of breast cancer.

Don't just go blindly surfing the Web for information on herbal cancer therapies, since many sites contain inaccurate information, making exaggerated and often misleading claims about cancer prevention, treatment, and cures. Commercial sites in particular should be avoided as they often make unjustifiable claims for herbal cancer cures, sometimes even promising a complete cure if you use their products. Think twice before using such information. Although evidence suggests that some herbs may improve a cancer patient's quality of life, others are dangerous and may be harmful. Get as much information as you can and always discuss it with your doctor.

One of the most widely touted herbal cancer treatments is Essiac, also sold as flor-Essiace, an herbal tea mixture developed by a Canadian nurse that claims to relieve the pain associated with cancer and even to reduce the size of tumors. Another is the Hoxsey treatment, developed by Harry Hoxsey and based upon a complex mixture of herbs such as licorice, red clover, burdock root, stillingia root, barberry, cascara, pokeroot, prickly ash bark, and buckthorn bark. Just before he died, actor Steve McQueen went to a clinic in Mexico for the Hoxsey herbal treatment (since the treatment is illegal in the United States.) However, there are only anecdotal reports indicating that either treatment is effective and no clinical studies to support their use.

Aromatherapy is a division of herbal medicine which uses fragrant oils from plants such as lavender to enhance moods and improve psychological health. These oils are usually used in conjunction with massage. Some reported benefits include an improvement in the psychological well-being of cancer patients by reducing both stress and depression.

The following Web sites have been created by leading cancer research and treatment institutions in the United States and should be the first place to go if you're looking for information on herbs and cancer.

Memorial Sloan-Kettering Cancer Center:
About Herbs, Botanicals and Other Products
<http://www.mskcc.org/mskcc/html/11570.cfm>

The Memorial Sloan-Kettering Cancer Center (MSKCC) is the world's oldest and largest private institution devoted to patient care, research, and education in cancer. The center's mission, the progressive control and cure of cancer, places it at the forefront of scientific research, as well as the development of innovative cancer therapies and new patient care programs. Though this site provides information primarily for oncologists and health care professionals, a consumer version of each monograph is available and can be printed. A useful FAQ section provides specific information on herbs and other dietary supplements, including which herbs might increase photosensitivity and hence should not be used when undergoing radiation therapy (see Figure 6.2).

M.D. Anderson Cancer Center: Complementary/
Integrative Medicine
<http://www.mdanderson.org/departments/cimer/>

Highly recommended. Affiliated with the University of Texas, the M.D. Anderson Cancer Center is committed to providing current information on all possible cancer treatments to its patients and the public.

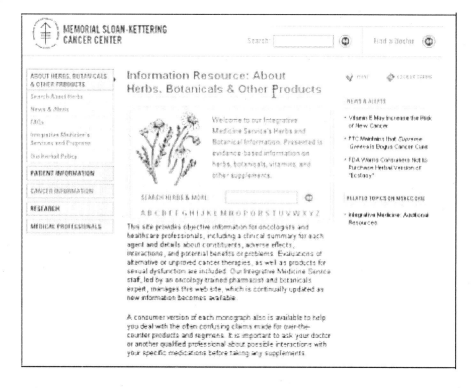

FIGURE 6.2. Memorial Sloan-Kettering Cancer Center: Herbs and Botanicals
<http:// www.mskcc.org/mskcc/html/11570.cfm>
Reprinted with permission.

This site provides evidence-based reviews of various complementary and integrative therapies, including herbs, and offers a glossary, a drug-interaction section, and links to additional resources.

MayoClinic.com: Prostate Cancer
<www.mayoclinc.com>

Prostate cancer is the most common type of cancer in men in the United States and the second leading cause of death in men. Several herbal products are marketed to relieve common prostate problems, including African plum tree *(Prunus africana)*, African wild potato *(Hypoxis rooperi)*, pumpkin *(Cucurbita pepo)*, rye grass *(Secale cereale)*, stinging nettle *(Urtica dioica),* chaparral *(Larrea tridentata),* and red clover *(Trifolium pratense).* What evidence is available suggests that if taken in small to moderate amounts these products appear to be safe, but up to now there have been no long-term trials to confirm their safety or to prove that they work. One herb widely used for "prostate health" is saw palmetto *(Serenoa repens),* which has been widely tested for its use in treating urinary symptoms in men with benign prostatic hyperplasia (BPH). Though it seems to be useful in alleviating BPH symptoms, it isn't yet known whether this herb has any role in treating or preventing prostate cancer.

MayoClinic.com is owned by the Mayo Foundation for Medical Education and Research, providing access to the experience and knowledge of the more than 2,000 physicians and scientists of the internationally renowned Mayo Clinic. Use the A to Z list of diseases and conditions to go to the section on prostate cancer.

Office of Cancer Complementary and Alternative Medicine (OCCAM)
<http://www3.cancer.gov/occam/>

Part of the National Cancer Institute (NCI), the Office of Cancer Complementary and Alternative Medicine (OCCAM) was established in 1998 to promote and support research in the various disciplines and modalities associated with the field of complementary and alternative medicine as they relate to the diagnosis, prevention, and treatment of cancer. Areas of interest include FAQs for cancer patients considering or currently taking CAM therapies, and links to fact sheets for cancer patients (see Figure 6.3).

OncoLink
<http://oncolink.upenn.edu/>

OncoLink is maintained by the University of Pennsylvania Cancer Center and offers in-depth online cancer resources for practicing physicians, and patients and their family members. OncoLink connects to the latest cancer news and research. The site is a little difficult to navigate, but provides useful advice on the use of herbs by cancer patients. To find information type your keyword into the Quick Search box.

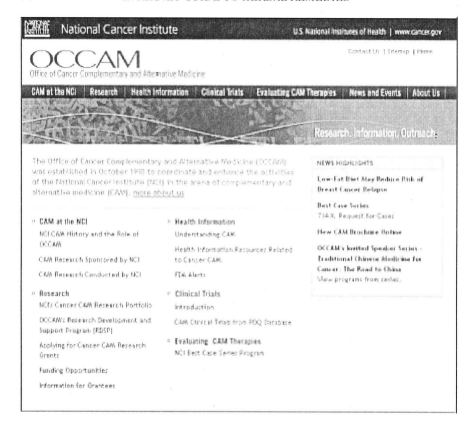

FIGURE 6.3. Office of Cancer Complementary and Alternative Medicine (OCCAM)
<http://www3.cancer.gov/occam/>

Dr. Susan Love: Herbal Remedies for Breast Cancer
<http://susanlovemd.com/takecharge/herbs_list.htm>

Dr. Susan Love is one of the pioneers and founders of the breast cancer advocacy movement. Her mission has been to encourage women
both to learn more about their own bodies and to become politically active to ensure that necessary federal funding will be allocated for research in methods of early detection of breast cancer. This unique Web
site for women provides up-to-date information on breast cancer, including comprehensive information on potentially useful herbs.

CARDIOVASCULAR SYSTEM

Clinical and laboratory research findings indicate that hawthorn (*Crataegus* spp.) may be beneficial in treating heart conditions. European studies suggest it may be useful for strengthening heart contractions, lowering blood pressure, and lowering pulse rate. The berries are widely employed for treating angina and congestive heart failure. Garlic *(Allium sativa)* is reported to have beneficial effects on some of the risk factors associated with atherosclerosis, in which deposits of fatty substances, cholesterol, cellular waste products, calcium, and other substances build up in the inner lining of an artery. Some claim that eating large amounts of garlic lowers your cholesterol levels, though it may have a much greater effect on your social life!

MayoClinic.gov: Garlic
<http://www.mayoclinic.com/>

Click on Drugs & Supplements at the homepage, then go to the alphabetical list under Supplement Information.

Dietary Supplement Information Bureau™: Hawthorn
<http://www.supplementinfo.org/aboutus/dsea.htm>

The Dietary Supplement Information Bureau (DSEA) is a partnership created to promote the responsible use of vitamins, minerals, herbs, and specialty supplements consisting of scientific, educational, and industry groups. At the homepage click on Herbal Remedies A-Z, then Hawthorn.

THE COMMON COLD AND THE FLU

Herbs such as echinacea, eucalyptus, garlic, and mint have been getting a lot of publicity as cold remedies. Echinacea is one of the most popular herbs in the United States and Europe. Several species of echinacea grow in the United States, the most common being the Eastern purple coneflower *(Echinacea purpurea).* The plant is part of the sunflower/daisy family, and its extracts have been used medicinally for centuries. It is widely used to prevent and treat the common cold, and is believed to boost immunity.

Common Cold Centre (UK): Alternative Common Cold Medications
<http://www.cf.ac.uk/biosi/associates/cold/home.html>

Affiliated with the University of Wales, the Centre is involved in clinical trials and basic research on new medications for the common cold. It provides much useful background information on the common cold, plus descriptions of conventional and alternative treatments.

Longwood Herbal Task Force: Patient Fact Sheet on Echinacea
<http://www.longwoodherbal.org>

An excellent review of the use of echinacea to prevent or treat the common cold and influenza, and the scientific evidence for its effectiveness.

DEPRESSION AND MEMORY IMPAIRMENT

Ginkgo is an extract from the leaves of the oldest species of tree on earth (more than 225 million years old). It is one of the most frequently used herbal products, especially in European countries. It's primarily used for alleviating memory problems but is also used to treat vertigo and tinnitus.

The most widely known herb for the treatment of depression is St. John's wort *(Hypericum perforatum),* with the bulk of evidence from ongoing studies suggesting that the age-old remedy is a reliable mood elevator for people whose depression is mild to moderate. St. John's wort is also taken to relieve anxiety, social phobia, seasonal affective disorder, and mood changes linked to menopause and PMS.

Studies also report the benefits of aromatherapy for relieving stress and depression. Aromatherapy uses fragrant oils from plants to enhance moods and improve general well-being. Essential oils are inhaled, added to water, or combined with massage.

InteliHealth: Aromatherapy
<http://www.intelihealth.com/>

InteliHealth has a well-written guide to aromatherapy and its uses. Go to the Complementary and Alternative Medicine section, then select Index of Alternative Therapies and Modalities.

NCCAM: St. John's Wort and the Treatment of Depression
<http://nccam.nih.gov/health/stjohnswort/>

The National Center for Complementary and Alternative Medicine (NCCAM) has developed this consumer fact sheet on the use of St. John's wort to treat depression to help consumers make informed decisions.

University of Maryland: Depression
<http://www.umm.edu/altmed/>

This site has comprehensive information about the signs and symptoms of depression, with links to fact sheets on St.John's wort, Asian ginseng, and valerian. Select Conditions, then Depression.

DIABETES

A number of plants with possible beneficial properties have been used in folk medicine and traditional healing systems around the world. For example, metformin, derived from Goat's-rue *(Galega officinalis)* is a widely used remedy in Ayurvedic medicine. Some evidence suggests that bitter melon *(Momordica charantia),* ginseng species, and fenugreek *(Trigonella foenum-graecum)* may be beneficial. Several of these herbs are used in Ayurvedic medicine.[6]

National Diabetes Information Clearinghouse (NDIC)
<http://diabetes.niddk.nih.gov/>

The National Diabetes Information Clearinghouse is an information and referral service designed to increase knowledge about diabetes among patients and their families, health care professionals, and the public. At the homepage select Treatments, then Complemetary and Alternative Medical Therapies for Diabetes.

Diabetes.1.2.3
<http://www.diabetes123.com/>

Diabetes.1.2.3 describes itself as "the world leader in online diabetes care," with information put together by an international group of pediatric and adult endocrinologists, diabetes nurse specialists, dietitians, exercise physiologists, and counseling specialists. This site has a great deal of useful material for consumers and health professionals interested in type 1 and type 2 diabetes. Under the Clinic section on the homepage click on Alternative Treatments. This is one of the best overviews of CAM and diabetes that I've come across, with brief information on fenugreek, bitter melon, *Gymnema sylvestre,* and other herbs. Also has a link to a useful overview of Ayurvedic medicine from the Agency for Healthcare Research and Quality (AHRQ).

Health and Age
<http://www.healthandage.com/html/res/com>

As people get older, their risk of developing diabetes (and other complications) increases. The Health andAge Web site is sponsored by the Health and Age Foundation (HAF), an independent, nonprofit organization promoting research into the aging process. For information on herbs which may be of value in the treatment of diabetes mellitus, go to the Alternative Medicine Center, then browse Conditions by Name/Diabetes Mellitus.

HEADACHES AND MIGRAINES

Migraines are severe headaches, which can be linked to food sensitivity, pollutants, menstrual cycle, or stress. They are associated with changes in tension within the arteries of the brain. Untreated symptoms may last for a few minutes or several days. Among the herbs known to have positive effects on migraines is feverfew *(Tanacetum parthenium).*

National Headache Foundation (NHF)
<http://www.headaches.org/>

At the homepage select Headache Sufferer, then select Headache Topic sheets from Educational Resources for information on feverfew and ginger.

Dietary Supplement Information Bureau: Feverfew
<http://www.supplementinfo.org/aboutus/dsea.htm>

At the homepage select Herbal Remedies A-Z, then select Feverfew.

IRRITABLE BOWEL SYNDROME (IBS)

Irritable bowel syndrome (IBS) is a disorder that interferes with the normal functions of the large intestine (colon). It is characterized by a group of symptoms such as cramping and abdominal pain, bloating, constipation, and diarrhea. Peppermint *(Mentha piperita),* one of the top ten best-selling herbal teas, is often used to treat symptoms associated with IBS.

University of Maryland Medical Center:
Irritable Bowel Syndrome
<http://www.unm.edu/altmed>

Select IBS from the Conditions section.

MENOPAUSE

See Chapter 7, "Herbal Information for Specific Populations."

PROSTATE PROBLEMS
(BENIGN PROSTATIC HYPERPLASIA, BPH)

Herbs such as American saw palmetto or dwarf palm plant *(Serenoa repens)* and the African plum tree *(Pygeum africanum)* are widely used

to treat benign prostatic hyperplasia (BPH). BPH is a noncancerous enlargement of the prostate gland, usually resulting in problems with uri-
nation.

University of Maryland Medical Center: Benign Prostatic Hyperplasia (BPH)
<http://www.umm.edu/altmed/ BenignProstatic Hyperplasiacc.html>

This site contains comprehensive information about the signs and
symptoms of BPH and links to fact sheets on relevant herbs such as saw
palmetto, flaxseed, and stinging nettle.

SEXUAL DYSFUNCTION/ERECTILE DYSFUNCTION

Erectile dysfunction (i.e., impotence) affects 50 percent of men age
forty to seventy in the United States. The public is continually exposed
to information on a variety of natural products claiming to restore erec-
tion and sexual vitality. What evidence is available suggests that most
naturally occurring compounds are not very effective. However, there
is some evidence that yohimbe *(Pausinystalia yohimbe)*, ginseng, maca
(Lepidium meyenii), and *Ginkgo biloba* may be helpful.

Horny goat weed *(Epimedium grandiflorum)* is a traditional herbal
medicine used in China (where it is known as Yin Yang Huo) and Japan. Although this herb has a history of traditional use for disorders of
the kidneys, joints, liver, back, and knees, its principle use is as an aph-
rodisiac. Legend has it that the name horny goat weed came from a
herder who noticed his goats becoming more sexually active after eating the plant. Unfortunately, there are no well-conducted clinical studies to see if it works in humans.

University of Maryland Medical Center: Sexual Dysfunction
<http://www.umm.edu/altmed/>

This site is a comprehensive source for information on all aspects of
sexual dysfunction, including male impotence, premature ejaculation,

and problems with sexual desire (libido). Select Sexual Dysfunction from the Conditions section. Includes information on dandelion (*Taraxacum officinale*), gotu kola (*Centella asiatica*), passionflower (*Passiflora incarnate*), saw palmetto, and other herbs.

SKIN CONDITIONS

Medicinal plants have been used to treat a variety of skin conditions, the best known being aloe vera for burns and wounds. Tea tree oil (*Melaleuca alternifolia*) has activity against certain bacteria and fungi, and is used to treat acne and fungal infections such as athlete's foot. Other herbs include vitex (*Vitex agnus-castus*) for treating premenstrual acne, and marigold (*Calendula officionalis*) preparation for the treatment of wounds, ulcers, burns, boils, rashes, chapped hands, herpes zoster, and varicose veins. Lemon balm (*Melissa officinalis*) can be used to treat minor wounds and herpes lesions.

University of Maryland Medical Center: Skin, nails and hair disorders
<http://www.umm.edu/altmed>

This site has a comprehensive overview of herbs in the treatment of acne, burns, eczema, psoriasis, and other skin conditions. Select Skin, Nails and Hair Disorders from the Conditions by Organ and Body System.

SLEEP AND INSOMNIA

Valerian (*Valeriana officinalis*) is widely used in Europe and the United States as a sedative and sleep aid. Studies suggest that extract of valerian root improves the quality of sleep, especially for those who are poor or irregular sleepers.

**ODS: Questions and Answers About Valerian
for Insomnia and Other Sleep Disorders
<http://ods.od.nih.gov/factsheets/valerian.asp>**

This is a comprehensive overview of valerian and its uses from the federal government's Office of Dietary Supplements (ODS).

*SPORTS INJURIES/
USE OF SUPPLEMENTS IN SPORTS*

Hoping to improve their performance, 30 to 40 percent of young athletes take a dietary supplement. Hundreds of products promise to build strength, increase endurance, burn body fat, and basically make us better athletes. Ephedrine, derived from ephedra *(Ephedra sinica)* (also called Ma huang), has been extensively promoted to aid weight loss, enhance sports performance, and increase energy. It also increases blood pressure, heart rate, jitteriness, and heart palpitations and may cause strokes or seizures. In 2003, Baltimore Orioles' pitcher Steve Bechler, age twenty-three, who had been taking ephedrine to battle a weight problem, collapsed and died during spring training. In 2004 the FDA banned the sale of dietary supplements containing ephedrine.

**Gatorade Sports Science Institute (GSSI)
<http://www.gssiweb.com>**

GSSI is a valuable resource for sports nutrition professionals, with articles written by qualified health professionals. In the Dietary Supplements section you'll find information about the dangers of ephedra and new, so-called "ephedra-free" supplements containing herbs such as bitter orange *(Citrus aurantium)*.

**InteliHealth: Ephedra (Ephedra sinica), Ma-Huang
<http://www.intelihealth.com/>**

A great source of information on ephedra, including news updates on the FDA's attempts to prevent its sale in the United States and easy-to-read information and warnings on its use. At the homepage click on

Complementary and Alternative Medicine, then Index of Herbal Medicines and Supplements.

SUBSTANCE ABUSE/ALCOHOLISM

Increasing interest has occurred in kudzu *(Pueraria lobata),* an herb widely used in Chinese medicine to treat alcoholism. Preclinical trials with kudzu have shown that increased consumption of the herbal formula is associated with decreased consumption of alcohol.[7] Extracts of St. John's wort *(Hypericum perforatum)* have been widely used in Europe for a long time to reduce symptoms of mild to moderate depression but recent studies indicate it may also help in reducing a person's alcohol intake.

GNC: Health Notes
<http://www.gnc.com/healthnotes/>

Go to the Health Notes Herbal Remedies section for a review of kudzu.

TEETH AND GUM DISEASES

Herbal remedies have long been used to treat both gum and tooth problems, though information is lacking on their actual effectiveness. "Oil of Cloves," from *Eugenia aromatica,* is widely used to treat toothaches. Some African tribes in Chad and the Sudan chew on sticks carved from the wood of *Salvadora persica,* or "toothbrush tree." Recent studies have discovered that *Salvadora* wood releases a bacteria-fighting liquid that helps prevent infection and tooth decay. It even contains fluoride.

GNC: Health Notes
<http://www.gnc.com/healthnotes/>

Go to the Health Notes/Health Concerns section on Gingivitis for information on herbal toothpaste and herbal mouthwashes.

URINARY TRACT INFECTION (UTI)

It seems that a glass of cranberry juice a day keeps urinary tract infections away. Cranberries *(Vaccinium macrocarpon)* have been used for the prevention and treatment of urinary tract infections for decades and were a widely used treatment before the introduction of antibiotics. Most women develop this type of problem at least once in their lives, and some suffer from constant recurrences. Studies suggest the juice contains chemicals which inhibit the activity of *Escherichia coli,* the bacteria most often responsible for cystitis.

Longwood Herbal Fact Sheets: Cranberry
<http://www.longwoodherbal.org>

An excellent review of the use of cranberry juice, with advice on its use during pregnancy, lactation, and childhood.

University of Maryland Medical Center: Cranberry
<http://www.umm.edu/altmed/ConsHerbs/
Cranberrych.html>

A well-written and detailed guide to cranberry and its medicinal uses with practical advice on its use in adults and children.

NOTES

1. Harnett SM, Oosthuizen V, van de Venter M. Anti-HIV activities of organic and aqueous extracts of *Sutherlandia frutescens* and *Lobostemon trigonus. J Ethnopharmacol* 96(1-2):113-119; 2005.
2. Ernst E., Cassileth BR. The prevalence of complementary/alternative medicine in cancer: a systematic review. *Cancer* 83(4):777-782; 1998.
3. Ernst E, Pittler MH. Efficacy of ginger for nausea and vomiting: A systematic review of randomized clinical trials. *Br J Anaesth* 84(3):367-371; 2000.
4. Seely D, Mills EJ, Wu P, Verma S, Guyatt GH. The effects of green tea consumption on incidence of breast cancer and recurrence of breast cancer: A systematic review and meta-analysis. *Integr Cancer Ther* 4(2):144-155; 2005.
5. Ha SW, Yi CJ, Cho CK, Cho MJ, Shin KH, Park CI. Enhancement of radiation effect by *Ginkgo biloba* extract in C3H mouse fibrosarcoma. *Radiother Oncol* 41(2):163-167; 1996.

6. Saxena A, Vikram NK. Role of selected Indian plants in management of type 2 diabetes: A review. *J Altern Complement Med* 10(2):369-378; 2004.

7. Overstreet DH, Keung WM, Rezvani AH, Massi M, Lee DY. Herbal remedies for alcoholism: Promises and possible pitfalls. *Alcohol Clin Exp Res* 27(2):177-185; 2003.

Chapter 7

Herbal Information
for Specific Populations

WOMEN'S HEALTH

The sexes in each species of being . . . are always true equiva-
lents—equals but not identical.

Antoinette Brown Blackwell

A growing body of research now points to significant biological and
physiological differences between the sexes/genders, with important
implications for the health care of both men and women. Women are
now recognized as having different health needs, different responses to
diseases, and different responses to medicines. As a result of intensive
lobbying from women's groups, research on women's health has mush-
roomed in the past two decades, producing a spate of books and other
information resources specifically addressing the unique health concerns of women.

The herbal literature is especially rich in remedies for women, probably because in many societies women have often cared for the physical complaints of other women, serving as midwives and often as the
community's chief healer. Thus there are many useful herbal remedies
for conditions specific to women's health, especially those associated
with the menstrual cycle, pregnancy, childbirth, and menopause.

Every woman will go through menopause. During this period of life,
most women experience symptoms that can include hot flashes, mood
swings, anxiety, reduced libido, and sleep disturbance. With increased

awareness of the dangers of using hormone replacement therapy (HRT), more women are looking to CAM for symptomatic relief. Five popular herbs used during menopause are black cohosh *(Cimicifuga racemosa)* and red cover *(Trifolium pratense)* to reduce hot flashes, St. John's wort *(Hypericum perforatum)* to reduce depression and anxiety, ginseng *(Panax ginseng)* to reduce fatigue and to increase libido, and *Gingko biloba* to counteract memory loss.

Dong quai (pronounced don kway), also known as Chinese angelica *(Angelica sinensis),* is an aromatic herb that grows in China, Korea, and Japan. It is considered the ultimate, all-purpose woman's tonic herb, and has been used for almost every gynecological complaint from regulating the menstrual cycle to treating menopausal symptoms. Because of its popularity I have included a link specifically for this herb.

The following Web sites provide information or links to resources for a variety of women's health issues.

American College of Obstetricians and Gynecologists: Herbal Products for Menopause
<http://www.medem.com/>

The American College of Obstetricians and Gynecologists (ACOG) is the nation's leading group of professionals providing health care for women. This ACOG guide is made available through Medem, a physician-patient communications network. To access the document, click on For Patients at the homepage, then Medical Library and Complementary and Alternative Medicine.

Dong Quai (University of Maryland Medical Center)
<http://www.umm.edu/altmed>

This site provides a comprehensive source of information on the uses of dong quai, including its use in the treatment of menopause and premenstrual syndrome (PMS).

SusanLoveMD.org: The Website for Women
<http://www.susanlovemd.com/>

Dr. Susan Love is a noted breast surgeon, an adjunct associate professor of clinical surgery at the University of California at Los Angeles, and director of the Santa Barbara Breast Cancer Institute. She is an author and patient advocate, well known for her down-to-earth style and ability to translate medical jargon into understandable concepts. Her Web site is focused on women's health concerns with an emphasis on breast cancer. As you might expect, there is much valuable information on herbs as they relate to women's health issues, such as hot flashes. Access the Complementary and Alternative Therapies section by clicking on the Take Charge button (see Figure 7.1). Under Herbal Remedies you'll find a list of herbs of possible use in alleviating the symptoms of menopause.

4.women.gov (The National Women's Health Information Center)
<http://www.4woman.gov/>

The National Women's Health Information Center (NWHIC) is sponsored by the U.S. Public Health Service and is a "combination Internet site/toll-free hotline dedicated to serving as a 'one-stop shopping' resource for women's health information." At the homepage, under Find Health Publications, select Browse Health Topics to go to an alphabetical list of topics, including herbs.

March of Dimes
<http://www.marchofdimes.com/>

The March of Dimes is a national voluntary health agency whose mission is to improve the health of babies by preventing birth defects and infant mortality. Founded in 1938, the March of Dimes funds programs of research, community services, education, and advocacy to save babies. This site has useful advice for pregnant woman thinking of taking herbal remedies for pregnancy-related discomforts—including information on herbs and herbal teas that should not be used during pregnancy. At the homepage click on Pregnancy and Newborn," then During your Pregnancy, and Herbs and Drugs.

SusanLoveMD.org
The Website for Women

home   decision making   living with   take charge

events   links   marketplace   about us

Dr. Susan Love Research Foundation

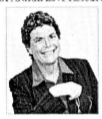

Despite over a decade of research, and more than $1.7 billion spent, 110 women are dying from breast cancer every day. Yet, we still don't know how breast cancer starts or how to stop it.

And we are still approaching treatment for breast cancer in the same ways: surgery, radiation and chemotherapy. This doesn't have to happen. The Dr. Susan Love Research Foundation is dedicated to ending breast cancer in the next ten years.

To learn more about the Foundation and how you can join us in helping to end this disease in ten years, visit our Foundation website here

DR. SUSAN LOVE
RESEARCH FOUNDATION

Wear Love!
Get the "Love" that can save lives. Purchase the Love's Army hot pink bracelet to support The Dr. Susan Love Research Foundation's efforts to cure breast cancer in 10 years.

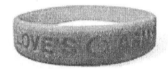

With the purchase of a Love's Army hot pink bracelet, you'll be funding innovative, fast-moving, leading-edge research that will eliminate this disease. I hope you'll consider buying a Love's Army bracelet and encourage your friends and family to also show their support. To purchase a Love's Army hot pink bracelet click here.

We are at the beginning of the end of this disease. All of us working together will have a profound impact. Join us.

Many Thanks
Santa Barbara Winery Supports Dr. Susan Love Research Foundation
Each year, Palmina Winery donates a portion of all sales of its Botasea vine to breast cancer

FIGURE 7.1. SusanLoveMD.org: The Website for Women
<http://www.susanlovemd.com/>
Reprinted with permission.

Longwood Herbal Task Force: Herb and Supplement Patient Fact Sheets
<http://www.longwoodherbal.org>

The LHTF Web site is provided by faculty, staff, and students from Children's Hospital, the Massachusetts College of Pharmacy and Health Sciences, and the Dana Farber Cancer Institute. Though primarily aimed at clinicians, the task force has produced a number of exceptional handouts aimed at consumers, each one having a short "Is It Safe for Children and Pregnant Women" section summarizing what's known about an herb's safety in breast-feeding and pregnant women.

Urinary Tract Infections (UTI)/Bladder Infections

Most women develop this problem at least once in their lives, and some suffer from constant recurrences. See the section on UTI and Cranberry juice in Chapter 6.

INFORMATION FOR CHILDREN AND PARENTS

The test of the morality of a society is what it does for its children.

Dietrich Bonhoeffer

Studies indicate that many parents give their children herbal remedies, such as chamomile, feverfew, ginger, and ginkgo. Unfortunately, there is a lack of good information available on how safe and effective they are. Some clinical trials, however, show promising results for the herbal treatment of specific pediatric disorders, such as extracts of kalmegh *(Andrographis paniculata)* of Ayurveda medicine for the prevention and treatment of upper respiratory tract infections (URTIs) and valerian in the treatment of sleep problems in children with an intellectual deficit (ID) (mental retardation).[1] Few parents or caregivers seem aware of the potential risks involving adverse reactions or dangerous herb-drug interactions.

Children are not little adults, and in the past have been harmed because of the lack of knowledge of how drugs might affect them. They have developing central nervous and immune systems that may make them more sensitive to the adverse effects of herbs. Children differ from adults in their absorption, distribution, metabolism, and excretion of drugs, and infants and young children are likely to be physiologically more vulnerable to certain adverse effects. Some herbs such as buckthorn *(Rhamnus cathartica),* senna *(Cassia angustifolia),* and aloe are known cathartics (i.e., laxatives), while some herbal teas and preparations such as juniper oil contain powerful diuretic compounds that promote the formation of urine by the kidneys. These actions may cause clinically significant dehydration and other medical problems in an infant or young child.

Parents considering giving their child herbal preparations should seek expert guidance first and make certain that any herbal preparations are bought from a reliable source, especially as a number of new herbal products specifically made for children are coming onto the market.

Longwood Herbal Task Force: Herb and Supplement Patient Fact Sheets
<http://www.longwoodherbal.org>

The LHTF Web site is provided by faculty, staff, and students from Children's Hospital, the Massachusetts College of Pharmacy and Health Sciences, and the Dana Farber Cancer Institute. Each patient handout has a short "Is It Safe for Children and Pregnant Women" section summarizing what's known about an herb's safety in breast-feeding and pregnant women.

FTC: Promotions for Kids' Dietary Supplements Leave Sour Taste
<http://www.ftc.gov/bcp/conline/features/kidsupp.htm>

The Federal Trade Commission (FTC) is responsible for monitoring the advertising of dietary supplements, in print and broadcast advertisements, infomercials, catalogs, and similar direct-marketing materials. The FTC's Consumer Education Office has developed an FTC Consumer Feature titled: "Promotions for Kids' Dietary Supplements Leave Sour Taste," which offer valuable "Pointers for Parents."

KidsHealth
<http://www.kidshealth.org>

KidsHealth is a popular site on the Web providing doctor-approved health information about children from before birth through adolescence. Created by The Nemours Foundation Center for Children's Health Media, it provides families with accurate, up-to-date, and jargon-free health information. KidsHealth has separate areas for kids, teens, and parents (see Figure 7.2)—each with its own design, age-appropriate content, and tone. There are literally thousands of in-depth features, articles, animations, games, and resources —all original and all developed by experts in the health of children and teens. At the Parents section click on General Health to get to the section on Alternative Medicine and your child.

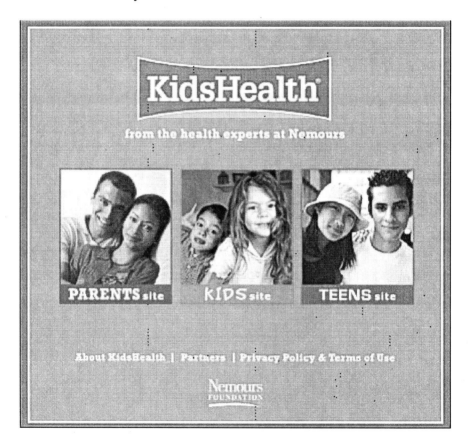

FIGURE 7.2. KidsHealth
<http://www.kidshealth.org>
Reprinted with permission.

March of Dimes
<http://www.marchofdimes.com/>

Though not specifically about children, this site has useful advice for pregnant women including information on herbs and herbal teas that should not be used during pregnancy. At the homepage click on "pregnancy & newborn," then During your Pregnancy and Herbs and Drugs.

AGING

Why should a man die while sage grows in his garden?

Medieval saying

As the number of aging/elderly increases in the U.S. population, there has been considerable interest in the use of herbal medicines to counter some of the problems many of us encounter as we grow older. The past few years have seen a significant increase in the number of studies conducted to understand how herbs might help slow the aging process. Some of these herbs are familiar, such as St. John's wort, ginkgo, and ginseng. Others are just beginning to attract attention, such as pigweed (*Amaranthus,* various species) to strengthen bones, and astragalus *(Astragalus membranaceus)* to strengthen the immune system.

A word of caution: some companies promote their products to senior citizens by making "anti-aging" claims for which there is little or no supporting evidence on their safety or effectiveness. Some of these products may cause physical harm, especially as seniors often have a high prevalence of chronic health conditions and take multiple prescription drugs, which increases the risk of possibly dangerous herb-drug interactions.

The following Web sites are designed specifically for seniors and their families. The Health and Age Web site is particularly useful for advice on which herbs you shouldn't take if you're being treated with particular medications.

Health and Age
<http://www.healthandage.com/html/res/com>

Highly recommended! The Health and Age Web site is sponsored by the Novartis Foundation for Gerontology, an independent, nonprofit organization. The Web site is intended to provide unbiased information directed toward the over-fifty-year-olds (see Figure 7.3). The Interactions by Herb or Supplement section lists herbs and supplements and the brand-name and generic drugs that may interact with them.

National Institute on Aging
<http://www.nia.nih.gov/>

The mission of the National Institute on Aging (NIA) is to "lead a national program of research on the biomedical, social, and behavioral as-

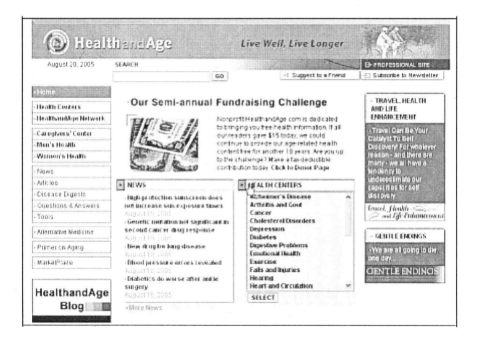

FIGURE 7.3. Homepage of Health and Age
<http://www.healthandage.com>
Reprinted with permission.

pects of the aging process; the prevention of age-related diseases and disabilities; and the promotion of a better quality of life for all older Americans." Go to the Publications section for documents on issues concerning the use of herbs and other supplements in seniors.

NIHSeniorHealth.gov
<http://nihseniorhealth.gov/>

This site was developed by the National Institute on Aging (NIA) and the National Library of Medicine (NLM), both part of the National Institutes of Health (NIH). It's designed to make aging-related health information easily accessible for adults age sixty and older and is also a useful tool for family members and friends who are seeking online health information for their older relatives. The Web site is organized by health topic. Each health topic includes general background information, open-captioned videos, quizzes, and frequently asked questions (FAQs). Though information on herbal remedies is limited, this is more accessible to seniors. For example, you can change the text size, change the contrast colors, or turn speech on or off.

NOTE

1. Francis AJ, Dempster RJ. Effect of valerian, *Valeriana edulis,* on sleep difficulties in children with intellectual deficits: Randomised trial. *Phytomedicine* 9(4):273-279; 2002.

Chapter 8

Herbs for Pets

We call them dumb animals, and so they are, for they cannot tell us how they feel, but they do not suffer less because they have no words.

Anna Sewell, *Black Beauty*

It's not just humans who benefit from using herbs. The recent revival of interest in "natural medicine" has moved to the world of cats and dogs. Spot and Fluffy are now getting the opportunity to try echinacea and ginkgo. CAM therapies in general are also becoming increasingly popular with organic food producers, partly as a result of a growing desire among the general population for more "environmentally friendly" treatments. In folk veterinary practice there is a long tradition of using medicinal plants to treat animals, where they're used with farm animals such as cows, sheep, poultry, horses, and pigs. Several currently used treatments for controlling parasites, such as mites, are based on compounds found in plants such as *Chrysanthemum cinerariaefolium* and derris root *(Derris elliptica)*. CAM is even used in the horse-racing world. Though acupuncture and chiropractic techniques are the most widely used CAM therapies for racehorses, since they help relieve pain and stimulate tissue repair, herbs are also recommended for a variety of ailments.

If Fido starts to look as if he needs cheering up, don't just start sprinkling St. John's wort over his food. It's important to remember that animals have very different physiologies than we do, so some compounds that humans can take safely can injure or even kill our pets. A well-known example is acetaminophen, the active ingredient in Tylenol, which humans can take with ease but which can kill cats. The use of garlic and other members of the lily family such as onions, shallots, and chives in a cat's diet is also not advisable since ingestion of these plants in a raw, cooked, or dried form can damage red blood cells.

If there's one consistent theme in this book it's "if you find information about an herb and are thinking of trying it, talk it over with your health care provider." Your dog or cat obviously can't do this, but you can. Pet owners should use herbal substances only under the direction of a knowledgeable veterinarian, who is familiar with the use of herbal preparations by pets. Much of the current use of herbs with animals is unsupervised, and myths and misinformation abound. Some products on the market have little or no efficacy, dosage recommendations may be inappropriate, products may contain harmful contaminants, and some contain substituted herbs instead of the ones listed in the ingredients.

Many Web sites offer information on the use of herbs in animals but there is little evidence that any of the treatments work. However, the following sites provide general guidance on their use.

equiworld.net
<http://www.equiworld.net/uk/horsecare>

Equiworld provides a wide range of equestrian information, horse links, equine chat, horse sales, riding schools, and lots more information. From the Horse Health section click on Alternative Therapies, then Herbs.

Veterinary Botanical Medicine Association (VBMA)
<http://www.vbma.org/>

The Veterinary Botanical Medicine Association (VMBA) was founded to encourage international interaction between veterinarians, herbalists, pharmacologists, and botanists to increase the safety and efficacy of herbal medicine use in animals. It encourages responsible herbal veterinary through research and education and increasing professional acceptance of herbal medicine for animals. The VBMA offers certification in botanical medicine and the Web site includes a directory of certified veterinary herbalists. Other features include a list of useful books and journals, practitioner handouts on "Herbs for Animals" and "Natural Flea Control," and a database of herbal studies in cats and dogs.

PetEducation.com
<http://www.peteducation.com/>

This is an excellent, easy-to-use site from two doctors of veterinary medicine (DVM), designed to educate the public about the health of dogs, cats, and other pets. At the homepage under Resources, go to the section on Holistic and Alternative Veterinary Medicine, then Herbs, Natural Supplements, Minerals and Vitamins (see Figure 8.1). This is a comprehensive collection of information on all the common herbs with useful information on their use in cats and dogs, for example: "Garlic at high doses can cause anemia in cats." There's also an impressive fact sheet on herbal adverse effects, "Herbal does not mean harmless" that you should read first.

The Veterinary Institute of Integrative Medicine
<http://www.viim.org/>

The goal of The Veterinary Institute of Integrative Medicine is to help integrate holistic medicine into the veterinary field. It provides educational resources for veterinarians and pet owners, including the Veterinarian's Desk Reference of Natural Medicines (VDR), which can be viewed online. Pet owners will find the VDR a useful source of information.

Whole Pet Vet: A Guide to Holistically Treating Your Pets
<http://www.wholepetvet.com/>

Provides information about acupuncture, gold bead therapy, chiropractic, diet and nutrition, and herbal medicine.

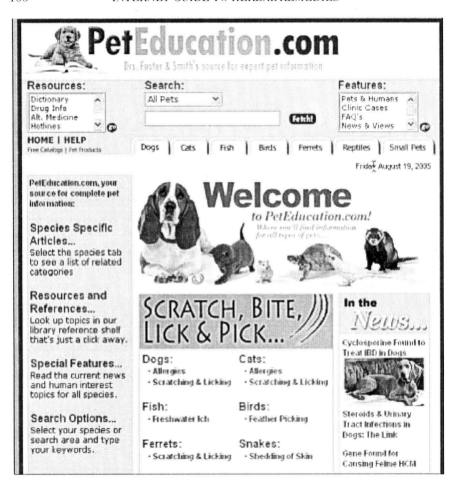

FIGURE 8.1. Homepage of PetEducation.com
<http://www.peteducation.com/>
Reprinted with permission.

Epilogue

The Bottom Line!

- Most of the herbs widely sold in the United States and Europe as capsules, tablets, and teas are safe if used correctly.
- "Natural" does not always mean "safe."
- Not everything you read on the Internet is true.
- Learn how to recognize a Web site you can trust and avoid sites that use words like "scientific breakthrough," "miraculous cure," "exclusive product," "secret ingredient," "anti-aging," or "ancient remedy."
- Make certain you tell your doctor about any herbs you may be taking.
- Be careful about taking herbs if you are pregnant or breast-feeding since very little is known about their effects on the baby.
- Do not give children herbal supplements without first talking with your pediatrician or other health care provider.
- Be very careful when buying herbs over the Internet.

Internet Guide to Herbal Remedies
© 2006 by The Haworth Press, Inc. All rights reserved.
doi:10.1300/5855_10

Glossary

adverse effect: An unintended effect of a drug on the body, usually unexpected. Some adverse effects can be very serious. *See* SIDE EFFECT.

allopathic medicine: The technical name for medicine practiced by MDs (medical doctors) and what the general public thinks of as conventional, mainstream, or Western medicine. It emphasizes the use of chemical substances (drugs), mechanical testing, invasive treatments like surgery, and a passive approach by the patient. This is a term usually used by alternative medicine practitioners: you'll rarely hear an MD describe themselves as an allopathic physician.

alternative medicine: *See* COMPLEMENTARY AND ALTERNATIVE MEDICINE.

aromatherapy: Aromatherapy means "treatment using scents." It's the use of pleasant-smelling botanical oils such as rose, lemon, lavender, and peppermint to improve health. It's considered to be a branch of herbal medicine.

Ayurvedic medicine: (Pronounced I-your-vay-da). An ancient system of health care from the Indian subcontinent. Plant products play an important role.

bibliographic database: *See* DATABASE.

blog: *See* WEB LOG.

bookmark: An electronic placeholder, like a physical bookmark, used to mark a location on the Internet. Web browsers can store and customize hundreds of bookmarks, a helpful way for people to organize their online interests and Internet research.

Internet Guide to Herbal Remedies
© 2006 by The Haworth Press, Inc. All rights reserved.
doi:10.1300/5855_11

botanical name: *See* SCIENTIFIC NAME.

botanicals: Medicines derived from plants.

browser: A kind of software that allows users to navigate the World Wide Web.

bulletin board: A bulletin board is an online message board where participants with common interests can exchange messages with one another, usually through USENET.

chat rooms: Chat rooms are exactly what they sound like—a place in cyberspace where people can chat and socialize.

clinical trial: An organized research study that helps doctors find out if a new drug, therapy, or device, helps, prevents, or treats a disease or condition. Clinical trials also help doctors find out if these new therapies and treatments are safe.

common name: The nonscientific name for a plant. Plants may have several common names.

complementary medicine: *See* COMPLEMENTARY AND ALTERNATIVE MEDICINE.

complementary and alternative medicine (CAM): A large group of healing philosophies, approaches, and therapies that are not usually taught or used in Western or U.S. medical schools or hospitals and exist primarily outside mainstream health care institutions. CAM may also be referred to as simply "alternative" or "complementary" medicine.

database: A collection of information organized in such a way that a computer program can quickly select desired pieces of data. You can think of a database as an electronic filing system. A bibliographic database contains detailed records and descriptions of books, journal articles (e.g., MEDLINE), or other documents.

Dietary Supplement Health and Education Act of 1994 (DHSEA): Legislation that laid the foundation for regulation of herbs in the United States.

dietary supplements: Products that include vitamins, minerals, amino acids, or herbs as part of their ingredients. You can purchase dietary supplements in pill, gel capsule, liquid, or powder forms.

eHealth: The use of computers and the Internet in the delivery of health care.

electronic mail (e-mail): A way of sending messages to other people in your organization or around the world using your computer.

electronic mailing list: A list of names and e-mail addresses of people who share a common interest and wish to communicate with one another. One e-mail address is used to send a message to all persons on the list. A program called a LISTSERV is used to manage this process.

emoticons: Symbols sometimes use in e-mails and chat rooms to show what mood a person is in. For example :-) means "I am happy" while :-(means "I am sad."

essential oils: Liquids extracted from the leaves, stems, flowers, bark, roots, or other parts of a plant. Used in aromatherapy.

Essiac treatment: Essiac is named after a Canadian nurse, Rene M. Caisse (Essiac is Caisse spelled backwards!), and is probably the most popular of all alternative treatments for cancer. It is basically an herbal tea, reputedly based on an American Indian formula.

FAQs: Frequently asked questions about a specific Web site and the information it contains. Read the FAQs first when you are new to a site.

favorites: In the Internet Explorer browser, a means to get back to a URL you like, similar to Netscape's Bookmarks.

folk medicine: Traditional medicine practiced by nonprofessional healers, often involving local customs or folklore. Generally involves the use of herbal remedies.

Food and Drug Administration (FDA): The federal government agency responsible for regulating food, cosmetics, medical devices, biologics (i.e., drugs derived from living ogranisms, such as vaccines), and blood products in the United States.

generally recognized as safe (GRAS): In the United States, the FDA classifies certain substances as "generally recognized as safe" for consumption which can be added to foods by manufacturers without establishing their safety by rigorous experimental studies. It includes many herbs and spices.

genus: (pronounced GEE-nus) A genus is a group of related or similar plants and can contain one or more species. A group of similar genera (the plural of genus) forms a family.

herb: A word nowadays used rather loosely to refer to any plant, or plant part, used for its medicinal or culinary properties.

herbalism: The study and use of plants for healing and the promotion of health. Often refers to a more nonconventional approach to the use of herbs for healing that includes folk and traditional medicinal practices not used by mainstream Western medicine.

holistic medicine: A system of health care that incorporates the physical, mental, emotional, spiritual, and social components of health with an emphasis on prevention.

Hoxsey treatment: Named after Harry Hoxsey (1901-1974), a self-taught healer who claimed to have cured many cancer patients using an herbal remedy handed down by his great-grandfather. Up until the 1950s, there were clinics in several states but after battles with the AMA and the FDA Hoxsey was eventually forced to close them. The only surviving Hoxsey clinic is now in Tijuana, Mexico.

integrative medicine: A broad, multidisciplinary, collaborative approach to medical care that blends mainstream Western medical treatment with complementary/alternative healing strategies.

Internet Service Provider (ISP): An organization that provides access to the Internet (e.g., America Online, CompuServe, Microsoft Network).

Latin name: *See* SCIENTIFIC NAME.

link, hyperlink: The connection between two pieces of electronic information or data. Clicking on linked text (usually underlined or marked by a specific color), or on graphical objects such as buttons, leads to another document or portion of the document, which in turn may provide further links.

LISTSERV: *See* ELECTRONIC MAILING LIST.

materia medica: A Latin term meaning "medical materials." Substances used in the preparation of medicinal drugs.

medical subject headings: Abbreviated as MeSH. Standard terms used to index journal articles in the MEDLINE database.

metasite: On the Web, a site that serves as a gateway to other sites on the same or similar topic. A metasite helps you get started in researching a topic. *See* WEB PORTAL.

National Center for Complementary and Alternative Medicine (NCCAM): The federal government's leading agency for research and education in CAM. Part of the National Institutes of Health (NIH).

National Institutes of Health (NIH): The NIH is a leading medical research center and the focal point for medical research in the United States.

National Library of Medicine (NLM): Part of the National Institutes of Health (NIH).The world's largest medical library and producer of MEDLINE.

natural: Existing in nature. Not a synthetic or manmade product, such as a drug manufactured by a pharmaceutical company.

naturopathy: A system of therapy and treatment that relies exclusively on remedies, such as sunlight, air, and water, supplemented with diet and therapies such as massage.

netiquette (network etiquette): Conventions that have been devised by Internet users for online politeness.

news groups: A topic-focused, public discussion forum on the Internet to which messages are posted.

nonprescription drugs: *See* OVER-THE-COUNTER.

not-for-profit: Also known as nonprofit. An organization whose main function is not to make a profit but to serve a public good.

Office of Dietary Supplements (ODS): A federally funded agency that supports research and disseminates information about dietary supplements, including herbs.

over-the-counter (OTC): Nonprescription drugs. Medications you can buy without a prescription.

PDF: Abbreviation for portable document format, a file format developed by Adobe Systems that is used to capture almost any kind of document with the formatting in the original. Viewing a PDF file requires Acrobat Reader, which is built into most browsers and can be downloaded free from Adobe.

peer review: Some journals use a board of referees to review submitted manuscripts to ensure that they meet rigorous academic standards of excellence and quality. May also refer to documents posted on a Web site.

pharmacopea: Also spelled pharmacopoeia. An official authoritative listing of drugs. Can also refer to a collection or stock of drugs.

phytomedicine/phytotherapy: "Phyto" is from the Greek for plant. Increasingly used in the medical literature to refer to herbal preparations.

plug-in: A piece of software that gives your browser extra functionality. For example, Macromedia's Flash is often used when viewing multimedia.

portal: *See* WEB PORTAL.

post, posting: To send a message to a newsgroup or other electronic discussion forum. A post or posting is the resulting message.

rhizome: A rhizome is a horizontal, rootlike stem that extends underground and sends out shoots to the surface. Ginger is a rhizome.

RSS: Stands for really simple syndication or rich site summary, depending on whom you talk to. RSS allows Web sites to automatically send regularly updated information to people who are interested in getting it.

scientific name: Also referred to as the Latin or botanical name. This is generally the most accurate way of referring to a plant. Many plants have similar common names but, by agreement, only one scientific name.

search engine: A search engine is a database that helps people find information on Web sites based on a keyword search. Google is probably the best known.

server: A computer that transmits or "serves" information to other computers called clients.

side effect: An unintended but known reaction caused by taking a drug. *See* ADVERSE EFFECT.

site map: A list or other type of visual representation of a Web site's content.

spam: Unsolicited commercial mail on the Internet, usually sent to newsgroups or via e-mail. Derives its name from a famous *Monty Python* sketch involving a group of Vikings repeatedly chanting "spam, spam, spam" in a cafe.

standardized extract: An herbal extract prepared so as to contain consistent levels of one or more active constituents. Standardization is the best way to ensure that a product contains what it's supposed to contain.

strobiles: Female flowers; conelike catkins. Hops are dried strobiles.

taxonomy: The practice of describing, naming, and classifying plants and animals. It was first developed by Carolus Linnaeus.

thread: A topic or subtopic within an electronic discussion group or forum.

Traditional Chinese Medicine (TCM): A system of health care based on the late-twentieth-century standardization of medical practices that originated in China some 2,500 years ago.

traditional medicine: A medicinal practice based on an individual country's culture, tradition, and customs.

URL: Short for uniform resource locator. The addressing convention used for all locations linked to the World Wide Web. Every "page" on the Web has a unique address, usually beginning "http://".

usenet: A network of thousands of topical electronic discussion groups called newsgroups.

Web log: A web log, or "blog," is what it sounds like: an online diary, in which the author (a Web logger, or "blogger") also links to other Web pages he or she finds interesting.

Web portal: A site (often a system) that creates a single point of access to information collected from different sources. A portal can offer a selection of resources and services, such as forums and search engines

Web site: A site or location on the World Wide Web. A Web site is a group of related Web pages. A collection of one or more Web pages on the same server, set up by the same author or organization, and usually on the same or similar subjects. One author may create any number of Web sites, and each Web site may contain any number of pages.

wholistic medicine: See HOLISTIC MEDICINE.

Wiki: Software that allows users to freely create and edit Web page content using any Web browser. Wiki is unusual among group communication mechanisms in that it allows the contributions to be edited. Not a recommended source of information for herbs.

World Wide Web (WWW): Popularly known as "the Web." Is not synonymous with the Internet. The World Wide Web is a means of accessing information on the Internet through a unified, "point-and-click" interface. The Web is based on http ("hypertext transport protocol"), which allows writers of Web pages to create hypertext links to almost any resource on the Internet, which people reading that Web page can then access by "clicking" on the appropriate hypertext links.

Index

[Page numbers followed by the letter "f" indicate figures; those followed by the letter "t" indicate tables.]

Acne, 81
Acquired Immunodeficiency Syndrome
    (AIDS). *See* AIDS/HIV
Adolescence. *See* Teenagers
Adverse Drug Reactions (ADR), 54
Adverse effects, 54
African Plum Tree, 72, 79
African Wild Potato, 72
Agency for Healthcare Research and
    Quality (AHRQ), 78
Aging, 94-96
    Alzheimers, 66
    dementia, 66
    drug/herb interactions, 94
AIDS/HIV, 66
    and St. John's Wort, 54
Alcoholism, 83
Allergic reactions, 54
Allied and Complementary Medicine
    Database (AMED), 50
Aloe vera, 40t, 91
Alternative medicine. *See* Complementary
    and Alternative Medicine
Alternative Medicine Foundation, 48
Alzheimer's disease (AD), 66-67, 68f
AMED. *See* Allied and Complementary
    Medicine Database
American Academy of Family Physicians
    (AAFP), 24, 55-56
American College of Obstetricians and
    Gynecologists (ACOG), 88

American Council on Science and Health,
    61
American Indian Ethnobotany Database,
    65
American Society of Anesthesiologists
    (ASA), 54, 55
Anderson Cancer Center, 71
Anesthesia, 55
Angina, 75
Animals. *See* Pets
Anxiety, 67
Apple®. *See* Macintosh computer
Aromatherapy, 71, 76, 77
Arthritis, 69
Astragalus, 94
Atherosclerosis, 75
Athlete's foot, 81
Ayurvedic medicine, 56, 65, 77

Barberry, 30
Bastyr University, 47
Benign Prostatic Hyperplasia (BPH), 79.
    See also Prostate
Birth control pills, 54
Bitter Melon, 77, 78
Bitter Orange, 82
Black Cohosh, 40t, 88
Black Current Oil, 69
Blog. *See* Web log
Blood pressure, 75

Internet Guide to Herbal Remedies
© 2006 by The Haworth Press, Inc. All rights reserved.
doi:10.1300/5855_12

Order a copy of this book with this form or online at:
http://www.haworthpress.com/store/product.asp?sku=5855

INTERNET GUIDE TO HERBAL REMEDIES

_____in hardbound at $24.95 (ISBN-13: 978-0-7890-2230-1; ISBN-10: 0-7890-2230-3)

_____in softbound at $9.95 (ISBN-13: 978-0-7890-2231-8; ISBN-10: 0-7890-2231-1)

112 pages plus index

Or order online and use special offer code HEC25 in the shopping cart.

COST OF BOOKS_____

POSTAGE & HANDLING_____
(US: $4.00 for first book & $1.50
for each additional book)
(Outside US: $5.00 for first book
& $2.00 for each additional book)

SUBTOTAL_____

IN CANADA: ADD 7% GST_____

STATE TAX_____
(NJ, NY, OH, MN, CA, IL, IN, PA, & SD
residents, add appropriate local sales tax)

FINAL TOTAL_____
(If paying in Canadian funds,
convert using the current
exchange rate, UNESCO
coupons welcome)

☐ **BILL ME LATER:** (Bill-me option is good on US/Canada/Mexico orders only; not good to jobbers, wholesalers, or subscription agencies.)

☐ Check here if billing address is different from shipping address and attach purchase order and billing address information.

Signature_____

☐ **PAYMENT ENCLOSED: $**_____

☐ **PLEASE CHARGE TO MY CREDIT CARD.**

☐ Visa ☐ MasterCard ☐ AmEx ☐ Discover
☐ Diner's Club ☐ Eurocard ☐ JCB

Account # _____

Exp. Date_____

Signature_____

Prices in US dollars and subject to change without notice.

NAME_____

INSTITUTION_____

ADDRESS_____

CITY_____

STATE/ZIP_____

COUNTRY_____ COUNTY (NY residents only)_____

TEL_____ FAX_____

E-MAIL_____

May we use your e-mail address for confirmations and other types of information? ☐ Yes ☐ No
We appreciate receiving your e-mail address and fax number. Haworth would like to e-mail or fax special
discount offers to you, as a preferred customer. **We will never share, rent, or exchange your e-mail address
or fax number.** We regard such actions as an invasion of your privacy.

Order From Your Local Bookstore or Directly From
The Haworth Press, Inc.
10 Alice Street, Binghamton, New York 13904-1580 • USA
TELEPHONE: 1-800-HAWORTH (1-800-429-6784) / Outside US/Canada: (607) 722-5857
FAX: 1-800-895-0582 / Outside US/Canada: (607) 771-0012
E-mail to: orders@haworthpress.com

For orders outside US and Canada, you may wish to order through your local
sales representative, distributor, or bookseller.
For information, see http://haworthpress.com/distributors

(Discounts are available for individual orders in US and Canada only, not booksellers/distributors.)

PLEASE PHOTOCOPY THIS FORM FOR YOUR PERSONAL USE.
http://www.HaworthPress.com

BOF06